PRAISE for
I Blew My Diet! Now What™

"If you've been struggling with improving your health, you can stop right now. It doesn't have to be so hard. Let this book teach you how to reclaim control over your eating habits once and for all using simple, proven tools that will change the way you think about dieting."

—**Mel Robbins**, *New York Times* bestselling author and host of *The Mel Robbins Podcast*

"A must-read! You'll delve into why you overate, find out how to reclaim your power, and discover delicious, healthy dishes to aid in weight loss. If you're struggling despite your best intentions, this book gives you the guidance you need to achieve success."

—**JJ Virgin, CNS, BCHN, EP-C**, *New York Times* bestselling author of *The Virgin Diet* and *JJ Virgin's Sugar Impact Diet*

"Normally diet books aren't my thing, but this is a health book like none other. Here you'll find out how to become the best you can be by goal setting, visualizing, engaging in empowering self-talk, and practicing gratitude. In between all the easy-to-read information, you'll find outrageously clever, original cartoons that invite you to laugh at yourself."

—**Jack Canfield**, *New York Times* bestselling author of *The Success Principles* and co-author of the mega-bestselling *Chicken Soup for the Soul* series

"This wonderful health book is delightfully entertaining (thanks in part to the cartoons) but serious enough to motivate readers to start new, healthier lives."

—**AJ Jacobs**, journalist, human guinea pig, and *New York Times* bestselling author of *Drop Dead Healthy* and *The Year of Living Biblically*

"Connie strikes a perfect balance between encouraging readers to be self-compassionate and find self-love while gently guiding them with proven tactics to become calmer and healthier and shed weight if that's what their doctor advises."

—**Katie Wells**, aka "Wellness Mama"

"Connie's book is a must-read for any parent who has had a love-hate relationship with junk foods, and who doesn't want to pass down that tumultuous bond to their kids. In these pages, you'll discover how to take back your power over unhealthy foods so you can reclaim the joy of eating nutritious foods in a way that serves you, your body, and your mind—and then teach your kids to do the same."

—**Elisa Song, MD**, integrative pediatrician and bestselling author of *Healthy Kids, Happy Kids*

"A truly one-of-a-kind motivating, mesmerizing, uplifting read!"

—**Debra Atkinson**, Founder of Flipping 50 and the #youstillgotitgirl

"This isn't just another diet book; this is a revolutionary guide that transcends quick fixes. You'll ultimately emerge healthier, happier, and more resilient."

—**Dr. David Friedman**, host of the nationally syndicated show *To Your Good Health* and #1 bestselling author of *Food Sanity*

"The reason why we blow our diet is not because we are weak. It's because there are many physiological dependencies created through food and habits that make it almost impossible for us to stick to a new way of eating unless we address the issues at the core and make deep lifestyle changes. This book will help you navigate through the emotions and changes you have to go through to find balance and control. It is written with love, understanding, and a nice touch of humor."

—**Dr. Anna Cabeca, DO, OBGYN, FACOG,** bestselling author of *The Hormone Fix, Keto Green 16,* and *Menupause*

"This groundbreaking book will revolutionize the way you approach what you eat. You'll learn that eating healthy foods is the fastest way to become your best self."

—**Mary Morrissey**, founder and CEO of the Brave Thinking Institute and author of *Brave Thinking: The Art and Science of Creating a Life You Love*

"It's exciting to see EFT's remarkable and proven ability to reduce cravings, enhance weight loss, and sidestep willpower discussed in this important book."

—**Peta Stapleton, PhD**, associate professor, clinical psychologist, EFT researcher, and author of *The Science Behind Tapping*

"A refreshing and empathetic approach to getting back on track with your health and reclaiming your power. As someone who has been there, I love how this book provides highly effective tools to develop emotional resilience and healthier habits."

—**Kristen Butler**, founder and CEO of the Power of Positivity, transformation expert, and bestselling author of *3 Minute Positivity Journal* and *The Key to Positivity*

"This pioneering book aptly points out that getting enough sleep is essential to shed and maintain weight."

—**Michael J. Breus, PhD**, author of *The Power of When* and *The Sleep Doctor's Diet Plan*

"This vital book underscores the connection between frequent drops in blood sugar levels and the onset of weight gain and metabolic disorders. Readers then get a tasty Bounce Back Diet that helps them balance their blood sugar levels and reach their optimal weight."

—**Keith Berkowitz, MD**, medical director of the Center for Balanced Health in New York City

"This book skillfully blends science with practical help, offering research-backed tools to help you rewire your brain, change your mindset, and regain control over your eating habits. A must read for anyone looking to make sustainable, positive changes to their health."

—**Srini Pillay, MD**, Harvard-trained psychiatrist, brain-imaging researcher, chief medical officer of Reulay, and author of *Tinker Dabble Doodle Try: Unlock the Power of the Unfocused Mind*

"As an avowed fan of body positivity, I'm wary of diet books. But Connie pulled off the near-impossible! She helps you shed weight for health reasons while you become friends with your body."

—**Jennifer "Jay" Palumbo**, freelance writer (*Forbes*, *Time*, etc.), stand-up comedian, and body-positivity expert

"A masterpiece that will help so many people! This book is not just about losing weight; it's about healing and making peace with your body. Highly recommended!"

—**Izabella Wentz, PharmD**, *New York Times* bestselling author of *Hashimoto's Protocol*

"Connie's book is a delightful read, filled with bite-sized, science-backed tips that can help you find emotional balance and sanity around food, especially when you're feeling tempted."

—**Tricia Nelson**, emotional eating expert and author of *Heal Your Hunger*

"Encouraging and empowering! Readers get simple, powerful tools to help weather life's greatest challenges, treasure their bodies, and eat healthy foods to lead their best lives."

—**Jennifer Joy Jiménez**, founder of the Health & Well-Being Division of the Brave Thinking Institute and creator of *TranscenDance*

"Sugar and carb addicts, take heart! This book is brimming with insights, success stories, and easy tools that help you turn your back on the toxic stuff so you can embrace a life of sweet freedom."

—**Michael Collins**, "The Original SugarFreeMan" (for 35-plus years) and host of the Quit Sugar Summit (11 years and running)

"Watch out for this female entrepreneur on fire."

—**John Lee Dumas**, founder and host of the award-winning podcast *Entrepreneurs on Fire*

"Connie takes a unique approach in this book to get readers to understand why they've gotten hooked on junk foods. She then empowers them to take charge of their eating using simple, science-based strategies."

—**Nir Eyal**, author of *Hooked* and *Indistractable*

"Readers will feel that Connie understands them and even reads their thoughts! This book will help you take back your power around food."
—**Jessica Ortner**, author of *The Tapping Solution for Weight Loss and Body Confidence* and host of the Tapping World Summit

"This empowering book brings hope and guidance to those who are stuck and wanting a healthier life. Well done!"
—**Dr. Tom O'Bryan**, world-renowned gluten expert and bestselling author of *You Can Fix Your Brain*

"This book explains why it's important to eat healthy foods to keep your blood sugar levels stable so you're happier, healthier, and more energetic."
—**Roberta Ruggiero,** founder and president of the Hypoglycemia Support Foundation

"I wish this book had been available when I was struggling with my weight! Connie writes with tremendous compassion, hope, and humor about the life-changing power of eating better."
—**Natale Ledwell**, bestselling author and co-founder of Mind Movies

"This isn't just a book; it's a beacon of hope for anyone who's found themselves at the bottom of a bag of chips, wondering where their diet plan went wrong."
—**Peggy McColl**, *New York Times* bestselling author of *Your Destiny Switch* and authority on manifestation

"A perceptive guide packed with effective, evidence-based strategies for people who overindulged in unhealthy eating. Wholeheartedly recommended."
—**Jill R. Baron, MD**, integrative functional medicine physician and author of *Don't Mess with Stress*

"It's fantastic that Connie shines a light on tapping as a rapid, potent way to change bad habits."
—**Mary Ayers, PhD**, psychotherapist, coach, and founder of Tap Into Action

"While you read this book, you'll feel like Connie is compassionately coaching you to break through to success."
—**Christian Mickelsen**, personal development and coaching expert and author of *Get Clients Today*

"I wish I'd had this groundbreaking book when I quit sugar and ultra-processed carbs 17 years ago!"
—**Sue Brown**, former sugar addict turned health coach

"Riveting, life-changing, and a major game changer."

—**Dave Asprey**, entrepreneur, *New York Times* bestselling author, and the "Father of Biohacking"

"This book offers a powerful roadmap to not only release those unwanted pounds but also to cultivate a mindset of resilience and self-compassion. If you're ready to break free from the cycle of overeating and embrace a healthier, more vibrant you, this is the guide you've been waiting for."

—**John Assaraf**, *New York Times* bestselling author of *Having It All* and *Innercise* and founder of MyNeuroGym, who shed and kept off 50 pounds for six years and running

"Kudos to Connie for showing readers how to eat better for the health of their hearts, moods, and bones."

—**Margie Bissinger, MS, PT, CHC**, physical therapist, integrative health coach, and bone health expert

"Connie absolutely nails it! If you want to be truly happy and healthy, you need to pay attention to what you eat and think."

—**Marci Shimoff**, *New York Times* bestselling author of *Happy for No Reason* and *Love for No Reason*

"This book is amazing!"

—**Cynthia Kersey**, bestselling author and founder/ CEO of the *Unstoppable* Foundation

"This book is a great resource to help you reclaim a healthy relationship with food and life. I especially enjoy its playful approach, extensive research, practical tools, and fun illustrations."

—**Laura Haver**, play expert and author of *Play Together: Games & Activities for the Whole Family to Boost Creativity, Connection & Mindfulness*

"A cutting-edge book that escorts you to take inspired action so you can become the best version of you."

—**Lisa Sasevich**, the "Queen of Sales Conversion" and author of *Meant for More*

"Bravo, Connie! This engaging, well-researched, conversational book will transform your life."

—**Linda Sivertsen**, author of *Beautiful Writers* and host of the *Beautiful Writers Podcast*

"This book is incredible! So good! This charming guide is full of fast, easy, effective strategies to help you get back on track after a diet setback."

—**Florence Christophers**, Kick Sugar coach and founder of the Kick Sugar Summit

ALSO BY CONNIE BENNETT

*Beyond Sugar Shock: The 6-Week Plan to Break Free of
Your Sugar Addiction & Get Slimmer, Sexier & Sweeter*

*Sugar Shock! How Sweets and Simple Carbs Can Derail Your Life—
and How You Can Get Back on Track*
with Stephen T. Sinatra, MD

I Blew My Diet! Now What?

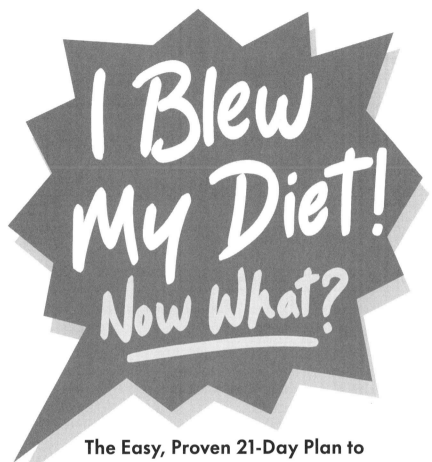

The Easy, Proven 21-Day Plan to
Drop Pounds & Bounce Back Boldly

Connie Bennett

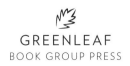

GREENLEAF
BOOK GROUP PRESS

I Blew My Diet! Now What?™
The Easy, Proven 21-Day Plan to Drop Pounds & Bounce Back Boldly

Greenleaf Book Group Press
Austin, Texas
www.gbgpress.com

MEDICAL DISCLAIMER
This book is not designed to, and should not be construed to provide medical advice, professional diagnosis, or treatment to you or any other individual. The information provided is not intended as a substitute for medical or professional care and treatment. Always consult a health professional before trying new home therapies, starting an exercise program, taking any supplements, or changing your diet. All information about specific foods, products, or programs has not been evaluated by the Food and Drug Administration, and any such foods, products, or programs mentioned are not intended to diagnose, treat, cure, or prevent any disease.

Library of Congress Cataloguing-in-Publication Data
Names: Bennett, Connie, author.
Title: I Blew My Diet! Now What?™ The Easy, Proven 21-Day Plan to Drop Pounds & Bounce Back Boldly.
Featuring The 21-Day Bounce Back Diet and the Bounce Back Boldly Plan.
Interior text design and book production services by Adept Content Solutions.
The Bounce Back Diet recipes and meal plan by Lizette and Geoff Marx.
Illustrations by Isabella Bannerman.
Cover design by Pete Garceau.

Subjects: 1. Lose weight. 2. Carbohydrates. 3. Keto. 4. Paleo. 4. Stress. 5. Sugar-free. 6. I blew my diet. 7. Fitness. 8. Low-carb. 9. Mindset. 10. Bounce back. 11. Bounce Back Boldly. 12. Tapping. 13. EFT. 14. Weight loss. 15. Release weight. 16. Body image. 17. Nutrition. 18. Health. 19. Crush Your Cravings. 20. Bounce Back Diet. 21. Visualization. 22. Positive Thinking. 24. Affirmations. 25. GoalPowerPlus. 26. Empowering. 27. Clean carbs. 28. Writing. 29. Hypoglycemia. 30. Low Blood Sugar. 31. Type 2 Diabetes. 32. Resilience. 33. I Blew My Diet! Now What? 34. Sugar. 34. Carbage (Carb Garbage).

Hardcover ISBN: 979-8-88645-280-8
Digital ISBN: 979-8-88645-281-5
Audiobook ISBN: 979-8-88645-350-8

Distributed by Greenleaf Book Group
To get special discounts for bulk purchases, please contact Greenleaf Book Group at (512) 891-6100 or orders@greenleafbookgroup.com.

Printed in the United States of America on acid-free paper.
25 26 27 28 29 30 31 32   10 9 8 7 6 5 4 3 2 1
First edition, March 2025

To you, dear reader, who—like me—blew your diet when you were knocked around by stress, heartbreak, or another major life transition.

May this book give you the hope, help, and confidence to discover why you overate, take back your power, and Bounce Back Boldly.

Contents

PART III: TAKE BACK YOUR POWER
THE BOUNCE BACK BOLDLY PLAN

Part I

THE PROBLEM:
We Blew Our Diets!

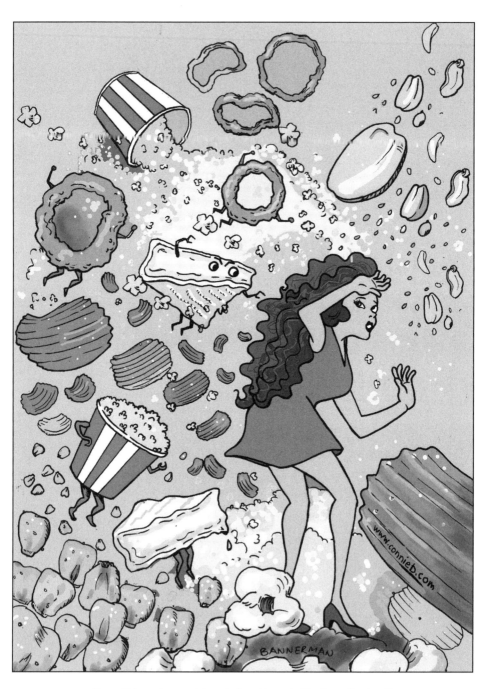

"Aaargh! I was harassed, haunted, and hounded by *Crazy Cravings!*"

Chapter 1

My Tale of Grief, *Heartbreak Bingeing,* and Triumph

Inhale the future, exhale the past.[1]

—Unknown

Excitedly, I reached the movie theater. I eagerly yanked open the heavy door. Expectation soaring, I stepped inside.

Then, I saw . . . *It*. My absolute favorite: Always-there-for-me crunchy, greasy, salty movie popcorn.

The mere sight of the machine spewing out mountains of the fresh, warm, yellow-white snack consoled me. The welcoming pop-pop-pop sound of cracking kernels made my weary ears rejoice. The intoxicating buttery scent soothed my shattered heart.

Suddenly, the most ferocious carb cravings pounced on me, seized control, and rudely shoved me into a mesmerizing concession area straight out of *Charlie and the Chocolate Factory*.[2] Yeah, I know. I'm exaggerating. Or am I?

Mind you, less than an hour earlier, I'd wolfed down a big dinner. Didn't matter. My already full—yet ravenous—belly demanded instant gratification. In that moment, I desperately *needed* the quick high I'd get from those oh-so-comforting carbs. Like a woman in a trance, I waited impatiently for my turn to order.

"A medium popcorn please," I anxiously pleaded.

"If you buy a large, it'll cost you just twenty-five cents more," the teen at the register nudged me. "Would you like a large?"[3]

"*What the hell*," I thought.[4]

"Okay, make it a large."

Carefully cradling the bucket of popcorn in my arms so I wouldn't spill any precious nibbles, I found and sank into a cushioned chair on a side aisle, far from other moviegoers.

Furtively, I crouched down, speedily shoveled fistfuls of the high-calorie carbs into my mouth, and greedily chomped.

I admit it. Very unladylike.

Within five minutes—before the film's opening credits rolled—I'd already demolished half the bucket's contents. In another few minutes, the rest.

When the movie ended over an hour later, I hankered for more munchies. Next, I drove to a nearby grocery store to grab and buy large packages of wheat crackers, sweet potato chips, and roasted corn chunks, along with a pound of rich Camembert cheese. Back home, I quickly devoured everything.

The Beastly Bingeing Blues Roared In

The morning after my gluttony, I felt repulsed by my ghastly behavior.

"#!★&!!," I angrily stewed.

"*I blew my diet . . . again!*"

Rage, regret, and remorse flooded my being.

Torrents of blame and shame—whose acronym, ironically, is BS—tossed me around like a small boat trapped by stormy waves on high seas.

Then, one persistent question ran loops through my brain like a rat spinning on a Ferris wheel: "How can I stop all this endless bingeing?"

Sound Familiar?

What about you? Have you, like me, ever felt so stressed, depressed, or outright "possessed" that you:

- Quickly stuffed your face with whatever processed carbs, fast foods, or sweets you could find?
- Started chomping on your favorite chips, cookies, or candy bar *even before* you checked out of the supermarket?
- Lingered long and longingly in front of your open freezer late at night while your family was asleep and then attacked that gallon of chocolate chip ice cream you'd stashed away just in case?

If any of those scenarios—or ones similar to them—ring true to you, then you totally get my previous plight.[5]

More importantly, the fact that you were drawn to this book means you're ready to end your self-destructive gorging for good. Hurrah for you!

Now let's go back in time again so you'll understand when, why, and how I blew my diet big-time.

I blew my diet! DEFINED

When I use the phrase "I blew my diet!" I'm referring to overeating high-calorie, ultra-processed foods that have been massively transformed from their natural state and then reconstituted in man-made laboratories by adding sweeteners such as high-fructose corn syrup and cane sugar, as well as salt, fat, fillers, binders, sodium chloride, taste enhancers, anticaking agents, emulsifiers, monosodium glutamate (MSG), and/or other additives.

Then when I say, "You blew your diet" or "You ate badly," I mean that you, too, overate unhealthy, fiber-stripped, unreal foods. Please note that I also use the word "diet" to apply to the way you eat as in, "Do you follow a healthy or unhealthy diet?"

Finally, "diet" refers to any meal plan you follow to peel off pounds or maintain weight loss. For the record, I'm against nutrient-poor, excessively low-calorie, or fad diets. Rather, I recommend the nutritious, blood-sugar-balanced Bounce Back Diet, which you'll find in Part IV.

My Tale of Three Moms

My dietary downfall didn't happen overnight. It had been brewing for more than a year.

First, my active, quick-witted, always-healthy mother was diagnosed with stage 4 lung cancer. It was clear to me what I needed to do. Since I was Mom's closest relative, I felt it important that I move from New York City to California, to be with her at the end of her life. This was doable since I was single and my own boss as a nonfiction author, freelance journalist, and health coach.

It took weeks—and many lively (okay, contentious) phone calls—to convince my fiercely independent mother of my plan to relocate for her. Eventually, she came round.

But when I rang her doorbell several hours before New Year's Eve—as we'd carefully planned—instead of warmly welcoming me as usual, my mother angrily kicked me out of her house.

I was shocked! Dumbfounded. Heartbroken. Who was this woman?

The nurse-caregiver helping my mother sympathetically shook her head and looked at me apologetically while she shut the door behind me. That was the first time I met the hostile, illogical, disease-ravaged version of my mother. Because she acted so strangely, I began to identify her as *Cancer Mom*.[6]

After Cancer Mom dismissed me and ditched our New Year's Eve plans, I whiled away hours weeping, wandering, and speedwalking city streets. Later, I grabbed dinner at a diner, stumbled onto a fireworks display, and ushered in the new year alone, while bracing myself for tough times ahead.

Thankfully, a few days later, my "second" mother, *Loving Mom*, showed up.[7] This gracious hostess urged me to leave the motel where I'd been staying and move into her house, as we'd previously agreed.

Loving Mom gave me towels, sheets, and closet space. She bought my favorite foods. She let me set up an office in her home gym. Now that was more like it!

Unfortunately, Loving Mom's warmth was short-lived, sporadic, and inconsistent. As the disease was invading her brain and body, Cancer Mom became increasingly angry, abusive, and argumentative.

Although I knew that the terminal cancer was to blame for my mother's excessive wrath and rancor, I still took it pretty hard. In retrospect, the meaner she got, the more I wilted.

I was always on high alert, scared that I'd do something "wrong," which, in her cancer-stricken mind, I often did.

In case you're wondering, my strong-willed mother refused chemotherapy. Instead, she chose to let the disease run its course and, in the meantime, she seized the day whenever and for as long as she could.

If you are or were a full- or part-time caregiver to either an ill or physically challenged loved one, you'll understand that I considered it my duty, honor, and privilege to be at my dying mother's beck and call.[8]

No matter how badly she treated me, I felt that I needed to be there for her. And so, I put her first, ran her errands every day, and did my best to cheerfully do her bidding.

Much to my relief, my "third" mother, *Brave Mom*, also started making appearances.[9] That impressive lady—the most fun of my three moms—valiantly squeezed out as much joy as possible as if from her favorite juicy blood oranges.

On her good days—when she wasn't suffering—my cultured, then-wheelchair-bound Brave Mom donned her polite party manners, and off we went to art films, plays, operas, museums, restaurants, and a nearby beach. Then on weekends, we hit farmers markets where she delightedly bought ripe plums, crooked squashes, and other delectable organic produce.

Brave Mom also made it her mission to teach me her favorite recipes. My best memory of our culinary adventures was the afternoon we excitedly prepared a soufflé. But just when we pulled it out of the oven, it collapsed into a formless, unappetizing heap! We laughed so hard that our stomachs hurt![10]

Another high point was the day Brave Mom watched me open a box of my then-new books, *Beyond Sugar Shock*, that my publisher, Hay House, had just shipped to me.[11] What joy it was to see her beaming so proudly!

But good times like that were exceedingly rare. On a typical day, my dying mother morphed from Cancer Mom to Brave Mom or Loving Mom and then always back again to Cancer Mom.

Suffice it to say that the unexpected was always to be expected.

Thankfully, a few days before her end-of-life transition, Loving Mom emerged one last time. After I tucked her into bed one evening, my normally undemonstrative mother tenderly told me, "*Connie, I love you very much.*"

To this day, I treasure those rare words of endearment from my reserved, stoic, European-born mother, who'd lost many relatives in the Holocaust.

You now have a flavor of the heartbreakingly bitter incidents and the wonderfully sweet moments that occurred during a time that I dub *My Bittersweet Last Year with Mom.*

After Mom Died, I Craved Carbs as Never Before

After I lost my mother, I lost myself. The brutal year with my terminally ill mother left me feeling bone-tired, broken-down, and brokenhearted.

The once calm, centered, composed Connie vanished. A sad, pitiful, powerless creature took her place.

All alone, far from my best friends and exciting life in Manhattan, I often sobbed in private, attended grief-support meetings, pounded away for hours on my computer writing early drafts of this and two other books, regularly saw a therapist, and, of course, hid out in movie theaters where I crammed down mounds of movie popcorn.

Clearly, my behavior around processed carbs was totally askew.

To be playfully self-mocking, I acted much like Pavlov's panting pooches, who perked up, salivated, and wagged their tails at the sights, sounds, and smells of tasty treats.[12] Go ahead. Laugh at me!

While movie popcorn was my hands-down favorite, I also went hog-wild over corn-anything, especially popped, fried, toasted, ultra-processed crunchy nibbles and other so-called *comfort foods.*[13]

Let's face it though, I didn't *really crave* carbs. What I *really craved* was my mother's unconditional love, approval, and support. Of course, that was impossible.

Although in my muddled mind, I gave myself permission to eat refined carbs, I still avoided sugary foods as I had for more than a decade. Strange logic, I know. Soon, I'll explain my twisted premise.

My Nicknames for Ultra-Processed Carbohydrates

Because all refined carbohydrates quickly turn into glucose in your bloodstream and then behave in your body similarly to sugar, I've created some easy-to-recall, catchy phrases for them. For instance, I alternately refer to nutrient-deprived carbs as *carbage* (carb garbage), *crappy carbs, culprit carbs, cunning carbs, fast carbs, junky carbs, much-like-sugar carbs, quickie carbs,* or *toxic carbs.*

Meanwhile, when I wasn't cavorting with carbage, I felt walloped by grief, had trouble sleeping, and was deeply depressed. Even more disturbing, I was haunted by flashbacks, hounded by nightmares, and easily startled. Later, I learned that those are signs of post-traumatic stress disorder, or PTSD.[14]

For months, my cravings for quickie carbs cranked into high gear, disabled my self-control, and shifted me into snack-attack autopilot.

Day after day, night after night, I mindlessly overate junky carbs in a fast, frantic, frightful manner that I now call *Heartbreak Bingeing*. (You'll learn all about this dangerous and widespread way of overeating in Chapter 9.)

After each binge, I promised myself to "eat right tomorrow." I'm willing to bet you've been there, too.

Usually, I began the day being "really good." For breakfast, I ate a half-cup of blueberries with two scrambled eggs and vegetables sautéed in coconut oil. But by late morning or early afternoon, my resolve inevitably fizzled, and quickie carbs called out to me again.

Soon, I was bolting down handfuls of the toxic carbs. Again and again and again…

As you'd expect, all those fattening snacks took a toll on my once-slender body. Within weeks, I couldn't squeeze into any of my clothes, so I bought one-size-bigger tops and sweatpants with an elastic band.

A few months later, my new clothes also became too tight. Again, I purchased larger, black, loose-fitting workout pants.

Finally, after I moved to a peaceful area some five hundred miles away from the plethora of painful memories, I was ready to find out how much weight I'd gained.[15]

One day, I mustered up the courage to pull out my bathroom scale. I stepped on it nervously. Slowly, I looked down. Within six months, I'd gained twenty-one pounds.

I felt utterly ashamed.

For Goodness Sake, I'm a Sugar and Carb Expert!

The reason I felt so humiliated that I put on twenty-one pounds is because I knew better. You see, I'm a recognized sugar-and-carb expert and author of the bestselling books *Sugar Shock!* and *Beyond Sugar Shock*,[16] which were endorsed by dozens of top health and wellness experts, including Dr. Mark Hyman, Dr. Daniel Amen, and JJ Virgin.[17]

In addition, I'm an experienced health and lifestyle journalist, a certified health coach, a life coach, host of my long-running *Gab with the Gurus* podcast, and the Sweet Freedom Coach, who helped thousands of people worldwide break free of their sugar or carb habits.[18]

But after that cruel year, Connie, the cheerful wellness expert, was no more. Frankly, I didn't recognize this woeful shell of my former self.

Even more mortifying, I'd already packed on ten pounds while my then-new book, *Beyond Sugar Shock*, was hitting top spots on Amazon bestseller lists in the United States, Canada, Australia, and the United Kingdom.[19]

It was impossible to escape the humbling irony: I felt like a Huge Health Hypocrite.

It Was Time to Take Back My Power

You know how you can wallow around in a dark night of the soul until you're sick and tired of being sick and tired and you've had enough already?[20] That's what eventually happened to me.

At last, one day, after months of hiding out in Heartbreak Bingeing, I resolved to get my act together.

The final straw was when my health took a huge turn for the worse. After I nearly fainted in a health food supermarket, I saw an integrative physician, who discovered that I'd developed insulin resistance, high cortisol levels, and adrenal fatigue. Later, I even got pneumonia.

My poor health, bulging body, and determination to walk my talk again catapulted me to action.

Suddenly, I was seized by a fiery, no-going-back, hellbent-for-glory commitment to put the kibosh on my carb habit, shed the weight I'd gained, and reclaim my good health.

As soon as I began to eat better, I began to think straight. Quickly, my insatiable curiosity was ignited, and Connie, the inquisitive journalist, sprang back to life.

My first order of business was to analyze what I'd been regularly over-eating to find out why I'd hurriedly packed on pounds without consuming one single bite of sugar.

I Tallied up My Intake of Typical Binges

Here are some startling facts I discovered by examining the food labels, ingredient lists, and websites of my favorite carb snacks.

- **Movie Popcorn:** Each medium tub of innocent-looking movie popcorn that I'd gobbled several times a week racked up roughly 1,200 calories, 60 grams of fat, 1,500 milligrams of sodium, and 83 grams of carbs, which quickly metabolized into some 20.75 teaspoons of sugar.[21]

- **Fried Corn Chunks:** Every four-ounce package of corn snacks that I nonchalantly inhaled added another 520 or so calories, 18 grams of fat, 640 milligrams of sodium, and 80 grams of carbs. On many days, I polished off two bags. When I divided the carb grams by four, I discovered that I'd been unknowingly stuffing down about 40 teaspoons of sugar at once, along with massive amounts of fat and salt.[22]

- **Sweet Potato Chips:** Even a large package of healthier sweet potato chips totaled around 960 calories, 66 grams of fat, 95 milligrams of salt, and 90 grams of carbs, which speedily convert to about 22.5 teaspoons of sugar.[23]

OMG! Those rough calculations made my head spin and my stomach turn.[24]

It was time to face the sour facts. For months, I'd been numbing out by carelessly flooding and abusing my poor belly and body with humongous amounts of toxic carbs, sugar, flour, fat, and salt. No wonder I'd gained weight so quickly!

Aha! I'd "Forgotten" That Carbs Are Like Sugar

As soon as I began to eat cleanly and, therefore, think clearly, insights came rushing in. One day, my intuition led me to look at my first book, *Sugar Shock!*, where I'd listed the forty-four symptoms (yes, that many!) I suffered more than a decade earlier.[25]

While I read, memories rushed in. There was the day I saw a new doctor to find out why I suffered from headaches, brain fog, heart palpitations, dizziness, fatigue (or the reverse, edginess), severe PMS, the shakes, crying spells, cravings, and other baffling ailments.

When my MD quizzed me about my typical diet, I reluctantly admitted to downing dozens of hard candies, sticks of red licorice, and/or small wheat crackers a day. Immediately, he knew why I felt so awful.

"You have low blood sugar or reactive hypoglycemia," he explained after tests confirmed his diagnosis.[26]

"To feel better, you need to eliminate sugar, other sweeteners, and all processed carbohydrates."

Sure enough, as my physician predicted, soon after I kicked all sweets and fast carbs, my ailments vanished, and I easily peeled off seven pounds to boot. Simply put, I felt reborn![27]

When I kept feeling great because I was well nourished, I became fascinated. My inquisitiveness led me to research and write my first book, *Sugar Shock!*, which educates readers about a constellation of symptoms (Sugar Shock and Carb Shock) suffered by millions, who often overload on sweets and crappy carbs.[28]

As I shared earlier, my follow-up book, *Beyond Sugar Shock*, was released while my terminally ill mother was hanging on for dear life.[29]

Now, I'm finally ready to come clean about the embarrassing timing as to when I blew my diet. A mere three months after *Beyond Sugar Shock* was published—while I was grieving, reeling, and struggling after Mom's demise—I was secretly stuffing my face with carbage after years of eating cleanly.

In short, I became much like you, the reader I now serve. That's why I understand and empathize with your predicament.

How This Book Was Born

When one epiphany after another hit me, it was obvious that I couldn't keep my many discoveries to myself. After months of mucking up my diet, I became determined to help you.

It was high time, I decided, to put my journalistic know-how, coaching prowess, and unstoppable curiosity to good use. At last, I became determined to learn from my many messes so I could share valuable messages with you.

My first mission was to find out why millions of us eat horribly when we know that we can do so much better.

Thus, this book began to take shape while I was reeducating myself about Carb Shock;[30] healing from trauma, abuse, and grief after my mother's death; becoming resilient;[31] discovering why I and millions like me overeat; shedding weight;[32] seeking and testing out powerful, fast-working, evidence-based tools to bring us back into balance;[33] and mapping out the transformational Bounce Back Boldly Plan.

Now, I'm so very happy and grateful that you're here. Welcome!

Look, I don't know the back stories behind your weight gain; the challenges, heartbreaks, or difficulties you've faced; or how long you've carried around excess pounds.

What I do know is this: bottomless bingeing and rapid weight gain are telltale signs of a life out of whack.

The good news for you is that you don't need to devote some seven years as I have to discover why you blew your diet, and then find fast, science-based ways to take back your power, crush your cravings, peel off pounds, make peace with food, claim calm, and step into an amazing life.

Yes, I did all the research and legwork for you. Let's just say that I took one for the team.

My Intentions, Your Intentions

Whenever we tackle a new project, it's invaluable to set specific goals. My heartfelt intentions are that this book gives you exactly what you need to reach your target weight and at the same time fast-track your happy, healthy, radiant life. Ultimately, by the time you've completed this book, you'll:

- Get a rock-solid understanding of 21 Reasons You Blew Your Diet and how you got to where you are.
- Learn practical, powerful, science-based techniques to self-soothe, give yourself lots of love and compassion, appreciate your amazing body no matter its present size, and shed excess pounds for good.
- Develop a good relationship with the healthy foods you eat and a hands-off approach to junky nibbles.
- Get original recipes and meal plans for tasty, nutritious, modified ketogenic dishes (KetoMod) so you eat well on the Bounce Back Diet while you take this uplifting journey.
- Find out how to unleash *GoalPowerPlus* (as I call it) instead of relying on often-elusive willpower.
- Pump up your motivation to keep the positive momentum going, and . . .
- Bounce Back Boldly[34] while you become your balanced, beloved, best self.

This is an uplifting time for you. It's time to get excited. Your bright future awaits.

Now I urge you to play full out. Let's get rocking!

Beyond-the-Book Support: Get Gifts to Enhance Your Reading Experience

While you take this transformational adventure to drop excess weight, make peace with your past, and Bounce Back Boldly, I'm offering lots of additional support. Sign up for your free book bonuses at www.BounceBackDiet.com/Book-Bonuses.

Chapter 2

You've Been Stuffing Your Face with Sugary, Fatty, Salty Junk Foods

Identify your problems but give your power and energy to solutions.[1]
—**Tony Robbins,** motivational guru and *New York Times* bestselling author of *Awaken the Giant Within* and *Unlimited Power*

For days, weeks, months, or even years, you've been a role model when it comes to eating clean.

You've been *that* friend, coworker, or relative—you know the one—who easily passed up donuts, French fries, and other fatty foods.

You've been so proud of yourself that you took control and made smart food choices. You made it look easy to peel off pounds—first five, then ten, maybe twenty.

You were getting more and more excited as you got closer and closer to your ideal weight. You joyfully imagined how great you'd look, feel, and act when you fit into your "skinny jeans."

But then *It* happened, and your world was turned upside down. Perhaps:

- A treasured loved one passed away—either suddenly or slowly.
- Your spouse came to you and said: "We need to talk." Before long, you were sitting in the law firm of "This is Mine, That is Yours" to finalize your divorce.
- You endured traumatizing emotional, physical, or sexual abuse.
- You've been a devoted caregiver to your terminally ill parent or child with developmental needs.
- You endured other adversities, challenges, or transitions such as a health crisis, accident, family strife, financial setbacks, political upheavals, racial unrest, difficult friends, or aggravating neighbors.

Let's face it, life throws us unexpected hurdles—sometimes several at the same time. All that can be triggering.

If you're like most Americans, when confronting life's lows, you've often found yourself face-to-face with a flurry of your favorite junk foods. Before long, you surrendered to that first bite.

Then one idea predominated. "What the hell," you thought. "I'll have just a few bites."

Uh-oh! That throw-in-the-towel attitude set you up for another high-calorie binge.

Am I describing your self-defeating pattern? What did you do when tough times struck, stress smacked you around, or your heart broke?

Like millions of us, you blew your diet.[2]

Admittedly, when hard times hit, a lot of people initially lose their appetites. But usually that doesn't last long. Sooner or later, many folks self-medicate with high-calorie desserts, crappy carbs, or fast foods. But, let's face it, over time, those unhealthy nibbles can wreak widespread havoc on our health, weight, moods, and life.

Hitting Rock Bottom Can Push You Forward

Now for the great news. There *is* a positive side to eating badly and packing on pounds. Yes, you read that right. Because you blew your diet, you finally feel inspired to give your body the tender loving care it needs. A wake-up call can take many forms. For instance:

- You get winded after walking only two blocks.
- Your favorite, once well-fitting dress, pants, or shirt are now far too tight.

- Your doctor warns that if you don't take off at least ten pounds, you may get cancer, heart disease, or type 2 diabetes like your relative(s) who died young.

All those scenarios—and more—can snap you out of your junk foods-gobbling status quo.

Turn the page. It's solution time.

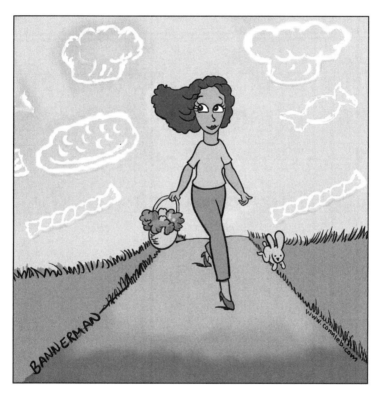

Bye-bye, cravings. Hello, happier, healthier body and life!

Chapter 3

The *Now What?* Solution: This is a Diet Book *and* a Transformational Guide to *Bounce Back Boldly*

Are you willing to design a future for yourself that demonstrates . . . that you love you madly?[1]

—**Lisa Nichols**, motivational speaker and *New York Times* bestselling author of *No Matter What*

As the title reveals, this book helps you release excess weight. But you'll learn to do much more than that. *I Blew My Diet! Now What?* is also a personal growth guide that shows you how to become your most awesome, bold, confident self.

To understand what I mean, let's look at this book's structure:

- In Part I—where you are now—you're getting the premise and the promise.

- In Part II, you'll do vital, far-reaching, life-changing introspection to discover 21 Reasons You Blew Your Diet.[2]
- In Part III, you'll go on the three-week Bounce Back Boldly Plan. That's when you'll learn how to implement Fast, Easy, Awesome, Simple, Tested Strategies (FEASTS) that nurture your body, mind, and spirit. You'll also be guided by a trait I call GoalPowerPlus instead of relying on often-elusive willpower.
- Then in Part IV, while you follow the Bounce Back Boldly Plan, you'll begin to drop pounds by following the nutritious, delicious, blood-sugar-balanced Bounce Back Diet.
- Finally, in the Conclusion, you'll get secrets from Successful Losers who've shed excess pounds and maintained their healthy weight for years. You'll also learn about the power of optimism, and you'll come to appreciate that eating nutritious foods is a safe superhighway to better health and self-love.

Peeling Off Just a Few Pounds Helps

Of course, you have your own reasons for wanting to release excess pounds. Whatever your motivations, you should know that even a modest weight loss of 5 percent to 10 percent of your body weight can lead to a variety of health benefits.[3]

Ample research finds, for instance, that shedding a few pounds may improve the quality of your sleep, reduce your risk of heart disease or stroke, lower your blood pressure and triglyceride levels, improve your mobility, and balance your blood sugar levels.

When you ditch extra pounds, you also may get more energy, boost your sex drive, and improve your moods. Just think: wouldn't it be nice to experience all that and more?

Take the Reader's Pledge

The degree to which this book will help you get the awesome body, mindset, and life you'd like is the degree to which you follow all recommended exercises and activities. That's why you'll now sign the Reader's Pledge to step up and give this program your all.

READER'S PLEDGE

I, _____ [insert your name], commit to learn why I blew my diet and follow the Bounce Back Boldly Plan and companion Bounce Back Diet so I can take back my health, power, and life. I now promise to:

1. Forgive myself for eating badly.
2. Stay curious and open-minded.
3. Carefully consider the 21 reasons I ate badly.
4. Test out all FEASTS (Fast, Easy, Awesome, Simple, Tested Strategies) and practice them as often as needed.
5. Give myself and my body lots of love, compassion, and forgiveness.
6. Put food in its proper place, which is to help me thrive and survive.
7. Activate GoalPowerPlus instead of aiming for willpower.
8. Test out the Bounce Back Diet recipes, eat all recommended, nutritious foods, and follow the KetoMod meal plan.

Your Signature

_____

(Date)

_____

WHY DOES THIS SERIOUS, TRANSFORMATIONAL BOOK CONTAIN QUIRKY CARTOONS?

Let's face it, those tempting ultra-processed carbs and sweets can take us over to the dark side against our will. When we're in the throes of Crazy Cravings, we may behave strangely (in private or even in public) and gorge on sugary, fatty, salty concoctions.

Years ago, while taking back my power after my prolonged fixation and flirtation (okay, addiction) to toxic carbs, it hit me that it would be a blast and give us much-needed perspective by politely poking fun at our collective plight. Since I'm not an artist, I found the talented illustrator Isabella Bannerman. That's when Sugar Shock Cartoons were born.

In between many laugh-out-loud moments, Isabella and I created the whimsical illustrations you'll find scattered throughout this book. Happy hunting! All Sugar Shock Cartoons are designed to playfully spotlight the sour truth. After all, as you've probably heard, "Laughter is the best medicine."

I invite you to get entertained now.

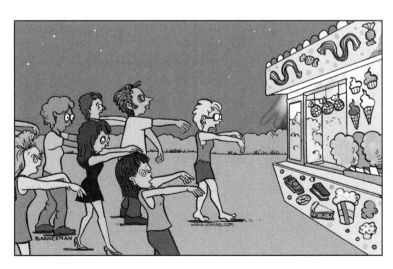

Are you a Sugar-or-Carbs-Craving Zombie?

You're Ready to Get Answers

Now I invite you to breathe a big sigh of relief. It's time to get educated, encouraged, and excited. You're about to finally discover why you blew your diet big-time.

Beyond-the-Book Support: Sign the Reader's Pledge

Download your Reader's Pledge at www.BounceBackDiet.com/Book-Bonuses. Print it out, sign it, and keep it handy while you go on this empowering adventure. If you like, keep your Reader's Pledge private. Or, if you prefer, share it with a friend, loved one, accountability partner, or success buddy.

Part II

Find Out Your Whys

21 Reasons
You Blew Your Diet

*I keep six honest serving-men
(They taught me all I knew);
Their names are What and Why and When
And How and Where and Who.*[1]

—**Rudyard Kipling** (1864–1936),
British writer

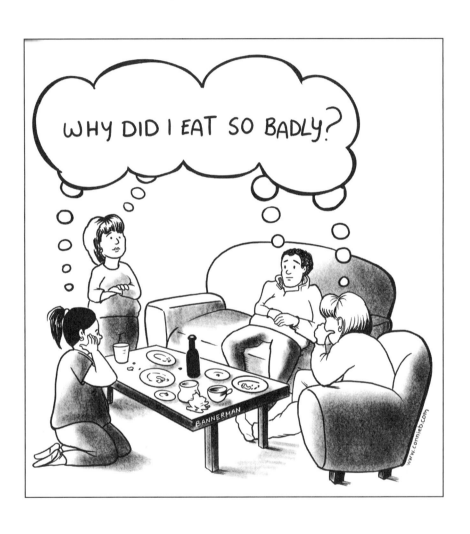

Chapter 4
Ask "Why?" to
Unleash Your Power

Regardless of WHAT we do in our lives, our WHY—
our driving purpose, cause or belief—never changes.[1]

—**Simon Sinek**, leadership expert and author of the *New York Times*
bestsellers *Start with Why* and *Find Your Why*

Why is one of my hands-down favorite question words. As a give-me-all-the-facts journalist and nonfiction author, I've discovered the eye-opening information you get by using that interrogative adverb.

Today, I invite you to think of *Why*—and its supportive companions *Who, What, When, Where,* and *How*—as your reliable partners that will help you finally get some answers to why you blew your diet over the years.[2]

In this section of the book, we'll explore a treasure trove of reasons—twenty-one in all—that led you to repeatedly overeat high-calorie sweets, quickie carbs, fatty dishes, or fast foods.

Let me reassure you: You have legitimate scientific, emotional, psychological, physiological, environmental, medical, or biochemical reasons for overconsuming junk foods.[3] That's right. In many instances, it may not be your fault that you overate nutrient-robbed foods.

Don't get me wrong. I'm all for taking personal responsibility. But as you'll soon learn, you're being endlessly cajoled, coaxed, and worn down by tactics that bombard you whenever you're out and about in a toxic environment I call the *Junk-Foods Jungle*. (More about that later.)

Let Calm, Creative Curiosity Guide You

Before we begin our introspective investigation into why you overloaded on high-calorie carbs or other unhealthy nibbles, you want to get in the right frame of mind. First, cast aside any frustrations, exasperations, or preconceived notions.

Next, calmly engage your inquisitive mind. Curiosity is a tremendous trait. It expands your mind. It prods you to find out more. It leads to many ahas!

Now invoke your creativity. Imagine that I'm your friendly fairy godmother waving a magic wand at you. Presto, you're transformed into your favorite fictional sleuth whose mission is to unearth answers about why you blew your diet.

Which imaginary detective do you like best? The brilliant, analytical Sherlock Holmes? The cheerfully astute, twinkly-eyed Miss Marple? The sassy, resourceful Veronica Mars?

Pick one of those private eyes or another gumshoe you admire. Now imagine that you're just as capable as her or him. Yes, you are.

Do the best you can until you know better.
Then when you know better, you do better.[4]

—**Maya Angelou** (1928–2014), poet, memoirist,
and civil rights activist

👃BREATHE, 🧍YAWN, 🎵PLAY PROCESS

Before we explore 21 Reasons You Blew Your Diet, you want to be in a state of serenity, acceptance, and objectivity. Here's an easy three-part practice to whisk you to this peaceful place.

1. **Breathe.** Draw in three deep, calming breaths. Slowing your breathing works magic. It helps you reduce stress lickety-split. It calms your nervous system, lowers your blood pressure and heart rate, and improves your concentration.[5] Indeed, slow breathing is "a natural Prozac," as pulmonologist Michael J. Stephen, MD, aptly put it.[6]

2. **Yawn.** Yawn three times. Mindful yawning is "the simplest, quickest, and most effective way to lower neurological anxiety in 60 seconds or less," explains stress reduction and mindfulness expert Mark Robert Waldman, coauthor of *How God Changes Your Brain*.[7] "It's one of the easiest and fastest ways to bring yourself into the present moment," he adds. "Yawning also makes it easier to identify important issues and find better solutions to problems."

3. **Play.** Finally, head over to www.YouTube.com to find the calming composition "Weightless" from the UK electronic trio Marconi Union.[8] This instrumental tune, which the group wrote in collaboration with Lyz Cooper, Great Britain's leading sound therapist and founder of the British Academy of Sound Therapy, was shown to reduce anxiety, slow your heart rate, reduce your blood pressure, and lower levels of the stress hormone cortisol.[9] *Time Magazine* even called "Weightless" "the world's most relaxing song" with "8 mins 10 secs of aural bliss."[10]

Sweet Success Story

For me, what's the greatest benefit of quitting sugar? Easy. It's the fact that I no longer feel any cravings for sweets or carby foods like bread. I've quieted that boring noise in my head about "Now, later; two, three; it's my birthday; it's special; more, more, more."

. . . I don't eat sugar, so those temptations vanish . . .

For me, it's so, so, so much more pleasant not to eat sugar! Someone said, "But where's the joy in life without the occasional brownie?" and I said, "Not eating brownies gives me more joy than any brownie ever did." For me.[11]

—Gretchen Rubin, *New York Times* bestselling author of *Better Than Before*, *Life in Five Senses*, and *The Happiness Project*

Final Steps before You Search Within

You have two last things to do. First, get a colored highlighter, pen, or pencil so you can mark sections of this book that speak to you.

Next, let your family or loved ones with whom you live know that you'd like some quiet time to explore why junk foods have held so much power over you. Now find somewhere you won't be disturbed.

Let's get started.

Beyond-the-Book Support:
Your Breathe, Yawn, Play Gift

To help you achieve a focused, receptive, serene state of mind before we explore 21 Reasons You Blew Your Diet, get my short audio download of the Breathe, Yawn, Play Technique. Access it at www.BounceBackDiet.com/Book-Bonuses.

Chapter 5

Why you blew your diet

You Were Tempted by Fast, Easy, Convenient Munchies in *The Junk-Foods Jungle*

> *What an extraordinary achievement for a civilization: to have developed the one diet that reliably makes its people sick![1]*

—**Michael Pollan**, award-winning journalist,
UC Berkeley professor, Harvard University lecturer,
and *New York Times* bestselling author of *Food Rules*
and *In Defense of Food*

Fast. Easy. Convenient.

Those three words sum up the dizzying array of nutrient-poor, high-calorie, ultra-processed snacks and meals that most people in the United States eat and overeat these days.[2]

Wondering what I mean? Let's face it—we live in a tempting, toxic Junk-Foods Jungle that relentlessly sets us up to cave in and gorge on a Standard American Diet, which many refer to as SAD.[3]

Coincidentally, SAD also is an apt word for how awful you can feel when you continuously ply your body with unhealthy food substances that are high in calories, artificial sweeteners, gluten, saturated fats, or chemical additives, as well as low in fiber, nutrients, and minerals.

In short, Americans typically load up on *unreal foods* that are manufactured in labs. These nonnutritive nibbles are the opposite of yummy, nutritious *real foods* that grow on trees, pop out of the ground, or roam on the range.

Knowledge is Power.[4]

—**Sir Francis Bacon** (1561–1626),
philosopher, statesman, and author

Ready, Set, On Guard!

In fencing, opponents use the term *en garde* [*on guard,* in English] to warn each other that a bout will soon begin.[5] From now on, I urge you to take this on-the-ready attitude whenever you step out into the Junk-Foods Jungle. Indeed, you always want to be alert to any threats to your health and waistline.

For guidance, let's get inspired by *The Art of War* from Chinese military strategist Sun Tzu.[6] Although this treatise is 2,500-plus years old, it still can help you face our modern-day health traps.

"If you know the enemy and know yourself, you need not fear the result of a hundred battles," Sun Tzu wrote.[7]

"If you know yourself but not the enemy, for every victory gained you will also suffer a defeat. If you know neither the enemy nor yourself, you will succumb in every battle."

The Junk-Foods Jungle

This is the toxic environment in which we live. The Junk-Foods Jungle is teeming with sugary, fatty, salty, fried, carbs-filled, ultra-processed temptations that entice you everywhere—in supermarkets, convenience stores, fast-food joints, movie theaters, food courts, office vending machines, and even hospital gift shops. This harmful atmosphere also follows you when you hop on the Internet, follow some of your favorite pop stars or social media influencers, and watch TV. But take heart. This book prepares you to become proactive rather than reactive to the fast, easy, convenient calls of the Junk-Foods Jungle.

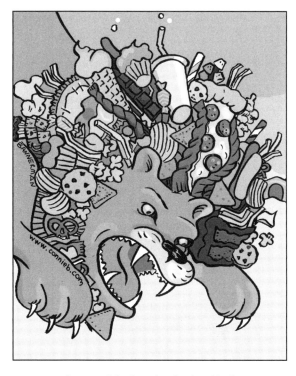

Beware of the Pouncing Cravings Lion!

Over Time, Our Foods Became Less Real and More Processed

How our diets have changed! Back in Paleolithic times, between about 12,000 to 2.6 million years ago, our prehistoric ancestors consumed only real foods—meats from wild animals and fish they caught, along with vegetables, nuts, seeds, or fruits they gathered.[8]

With the advent of the Industrial Revolution nearly 300 years ago, companies began to mechanize food production.[9] Over time, processing became faster, more extensive, and increasingly complicated as sweeteners, preservatives, flavor enhancers, stabilizers, solvents, binders, bulking agents, colors, and salt were added to enhance texture, increase palatability, and extend the shelf life of ultra-processed foods.[10]

The result? A preponderance of fake, manufactured foods that bear little resemblance to the natural foods from which they were derived.

"Our diets have changed more in the last century than in the previous 10,000 years," points out Melanie Warner, author of *Pandora's Lunchbox: How Processed Food Took Over the American Meal.*[11]

"The avalanche of prefabbed, precooked, often portable food into every corner of American society represents the most dramatic nutritional shift in human history," explained Warner, a former *New York Times* reporter.

This unhealthy trend is still going strong. Americans get about 80 percent of their total calories from ultra-processed foods and beverages that are high in energy, saturated fat, sugar, and salt.

"The US packaged food and beverage supply is . . . highly processed, and generally unhealthy," a study in *Nutrients* revealed.[12]

To arrive at these findings, the researchers examined more than 230,000 products that play "a central role in the development of chronic disease, including obesity and cardiovascular disease."

If you put junk food in your body,
your body will turn to junk.[13]

—Goldie Hawn,
Academy Award-winning actress

America, the Land of the Obese and the Home of the Mostly Overweight

Although this is intended to be a hopeful, helpful book, we need to consider where we are as a nation and world when it comes to our weight. Nearly three-quarters of American adults over age twenty are now either overweight or obese, according to the Centers for Disease Control and Prevention (CDC).[14] That comes to about 139 million obese adults and 100 million overweight adults in the United States.

America isn't the only country facing widespread weight gain. "Worldwide obesity has nearly tripled since 1975," points out the World Health Organization (WHO), which classifies obesity as a "predictable and preventable health crisis."[15]

Across the globe, more than 1.9 billion adults aged eighteen and older and over 340 million children and adolescents aged five to nineteen are overweight or obese, according to the WHO.

Why is it so important to let go of excess weight? Research reveals that people who are obese or overweight are at greater risk for a host of health problems, including high blood pressure (hypertension), type 2 diabetes, coronary heart disease, stroke, gallbladder disease, high LDL (the bad) cholesterol, various cancers, and high levels of triglycerides.[16]

But the good news is that you're now here to set in motion plans to become healthier.

Do You Take the Fast, Easy, Convenient Route?

Let's now look at your typical patterns to discover how often you grab and eat unhealthy junk foods that may lead to weight gain. Think about your routine when you're out and about in the Junk-Foods Jungle.[17] Do you:

- Start your day hurriedly polishing off a large bowl of cold cereal topped with milk and sugar, a waffle drenched in rich syrup, and/or a slice of toast slathered with gobs of butter and jam?
- Skip a healthy breakfast and instead slug down a sweetened, calorie-loaded, whipped cream–laden coffee beverage and get a sweet roll or chocolate–glazed donut while on the run?
- Grab a hamburger on a white-flour bun for lunch at a fast-food joint; spread it with heaps of sugar-filled ketchup, fatty mayo, salty

pickles; and then top off your meal with French fries, a milk shake, and/or a piece of apple pie?

- Mindlessly snack at your desk on handfuls of potato chips, chocolate-covered nuts, or granola bars?
- Regularly gulp down sugar-filled soda, fruit drinks, sports or energy beverages, or sweetened coffee or tea?
- Often order fattening ready-made meals for dinner like pizza, submarine sandwiches, or fried chicken with cornbread?

Now consider your routines. Do you frequently inhale fast, easy, convenient junk food munchies? If that's the case, check yes next to Reason #1 on your 21 Reasons I Blew My Diet List. (See below to find out how to get it.)

Beyond-the-Book Support: Get Your 21 Reasons List to Keep Track While You Read

To remember 21 Reasons You Blew Your Diet, print out the download provided, keep it handy while we dig deeper in Part II (through Chapter 17), and check off those reasons that apply to you. Access it at <u>www.BounceBackDiet.com/Book-Bonuses</u>.

Chapter 6

Why you blew your diet

Your Binge-Watching Prompted *Binge-Snacking, See-It-Crave-It Gorging,* or *Late-Night Grazing*

[TV ads prime] you to seek out ultra-processed foods. So, you'll start scrounging around in your kitchen, and you might not even make the link between what you've seen on the TV and why you suddenly have a hankering for food. It's not ... about needing calories; it's about desiring the reward of the food.[1]

—**Ashley Gearhardt, PhD**, psychology professor at the University of Michigan and director of its Food and Addiction Science and Treatment (FAST) Lab

You and your sweetheart are curled up on the couch in front of your television to binge-watch your favorite show. It's getting late and you really should go to bed, but you want to find out what happens next.

"Just one more episode," you and your honey decide. But when that episode is over, you keep watching. Another 45 minutes or so later, you still don't turn off the tube to catch yet another episode. Ring a bell?

Whatever program you turn on in any genre—whether it's action, adventure, romantic comedy, medical drama, science fiction, or historical thriller—the results are likely the same.

While you're catching the plot's twists and turns *on screen*, you're paying little attention to what you're doing *off screen*, and that's when you may unthinkingly grab and gobble sweets, fast foods, or carb munchies.

The upshot: While you're binge-watching your favorite streamed or TV shows, you also may do binge-snacking.

As Binge-Watching Soars, So Does Binge-Snacking

These days, about 73 percent of US adults binge-watch two to six episodes of a favorite streamed show in one sitting, according to a Deloitte Digital Democracy survey.[2]

In fact, streaming content has now overtaken live programming as the method most people prefer.

The explosion of binge-watching has led health experts to caution that frittering away many hours in front of the screen may increase the risk for such health conditions as heart disease, sleep problems, depression, and even behavioral addictions.

Researchers also are concerned that long screen time may lead people to exercise less, become socially isolated, and even develop cognitive decline over time.[3]

Not only that, but settling in for marathon viewing sessions can lead to unhealthy eating patterns such as consuming lots of junk foods and mindlessly snacking in front of your screen.

Research in *BMC Public Health* found that poor dietary choices seem connected to extended use of screen-based devices, especially TVs and smartphones.[4] Heavy and moderate users of screens reported higher body mass index (BMI) scores compared to light users.

Binge Snacking and See-It-Crave-It Gorging

When you watch movies or binge-watch two or more episodes of streaming or television shows on your TV, laptop, tablet, or phone, you may do what I dub Binge Snacking. (That's when you consume so much food that it's like a binge.)

In addition, after you see unhealthy foods and drinks advertised, your desire for them increases, and you may do two other kinds of overeating, which I call See-It-Crave-It Gorging and Late-Night Grazing. (More later about the latter.)

How You're Being Seduced to Indulge When You Stream or Watch Movies

When you're binge-watching your favorite series on your favorite streaming platform, you're influenced in your buying and consuming decisions by the practice of *embedded marketing,* better known as product placement.[5]

Now a $23 billion industry, product placement is when companies work in concert with content creators to put their products into the plot or set of a TV show, movie, or music video.[6]

"Streaming fans, let it be known: You will be marketed to. Somehow, some way," *Forbes* contributor Andy Meek cautioned in his article, "Brands Are Invading Your Favorite Streaming Shows and Movies, Whether You Realize It or Not."[7]

Meanwhile, most films depicted people eating "mostly unhealthy" diets high in sugar and alcohol, according to a study in *JAMA Internal Medicine* from Stanford University psychologists, who looked at the 250 top-grossing Hollywood movies between 1994 and 2018.[8]

"The foods depicted in popular movies send a clear message—not only about what is common to eat but also about what foods are appealing or cool to eat," said Alia Crum, PhD, assistant professor of psychology and senior author of the study. "If our favorite actors and superheroes aren't eating salads, why should we?"[9]

Celebrity-Driven Advertising Contributes to the Obesity Epidemic

Meanwhile, every time you turn on the tube, get on the Internet, or attend major outdoor events, you'll likely be subtly prodded by celebrities or influencers who cheerfully invite you to consume various unhealthy junk foods and beverages.[10]

You're seeing these star-studded ads, because top pop stars, rappers, athletes, or influencers have inked incredibly lucrative endorsement deals with processed food companies that seek to reach millions of their fans.

An estimated 80.8 percent of endorsed foods were nutrient poor and energy dense (sweets, processed carbs, and deep-fried foods that are high in calories), and 71 percent of nonalcoholic beverages were sugar-sweetened, according to a study in *Pediatrics*.[11]

Frankly, I find the phenomenon of celebrity junk-food endorsements alarming. Whenever influencers promote certain ultra-processed snacks, meals, or beverages, millions of their adoring fans—often unsuspecting children and teens—may follow their unhealthy examples without giving it any thought. Devotees may unthinkingly assume that if so-and-so star recommends XYZ product, they should buy it.

Let me be blunt here. When big names endorse sugar-filled drinks or high-calorie, carb-rich snacks, they're recommending unhealthy eating behaviors which can perpetuate the obesity crisis.[12]

Food, beverage, and restaurant companies spend almost $14 billion each year on advertising in the United States. More than 80 percent of that ad budget, or about $11 billion, goes to promote fast food, sugary drinks, candy, and unhealthy snacks, according to an analysis of Nielsen data from the UConn Rudd Center for Food Policy and Health.[13]

Beverage companies allocated over $1 billion to advertise sugary and energy drinks in 2018, according to Sugary Drinks FACTS 2020, a report from the Rudd Center.[14]

Incidentally, the entire budget for all chronic disease prevention and health promotion at the CDC is also $1 billion.

There's convincing evidence in adults that the more television they watch, the more likely they are to gain weight or become overweight or obese. TV viewing may also promote poor dietary behavior due to frequent exposure to unhealthy food and beverage marketing, as well as providing more opportunities for unhealthy snacking, and interfering with adequate sleep.[15]

—**Lilian Cheung,** DSc, director of health promotion and communication at the Harvard T. H. Chan School of Public Health, and coauthor of *Savor: Mindful Eating, Mindful Life* with the late Buddhist monk and Zen master **Thich Nhất Hanh**

Advertising on TV, Movies, or the Internet May Lead to See-It-Crave-It Gorging

How can food advertisements entice you to overeat? Ads may provocatively and glamorously portray what has been referred to as *gastro-porn* or *food porn*.[16] Let's look at some alarming findings:

- **Just seeing pictures of food can stimulate eating and weight gain.** Yale University scientists analyzed data from nearly 3,300 participants and discovered that looking at pictures or videos of food was *just as* likely to cause people to reach for something unhealthy to eat as being tempted by those junk foods in real life. Interestingly, seeing pictures caused *more* cravings than smelling the actual foods. The research, which was published in *Obesity Reviews*, also discovered that these folks were *more* apt to gain weight in a two-year study follow-up.[17]

- **Visual cues can make you eat more.** A study published in *Clinical Psychological Science* confirmed that visual, auditory, and olfactory (sight, sound, smell) stimulation can prompt you to eat more than if you're in a *noncue* environment. Researchers found that when surrounded by the aromas, menu signage, and background music typically found at fast food restaurants, people ate 220 more calories. They didn't report liking the foods anymore; they just felt hungrier and wanted them more.[18]

- **Hunger hormones are triggered by food pictures.** Seeing pictures of food may cause an upswing in levels of *ghrelin* ("the hunger hormone"), which stimulates appetite, increases food intake, and promotes fat storage, according to a study published in the journal *PLOS One.* Subjects liked pictures of desserts and sweets more than those of protein-rich meats, fish, and meat-based fast foods and felt hungrier after viewing the sweets.[19]

Avoid foods you see
advertised on television.[20]

—**Michael Pollan**,
author of *Food Rules*

Can Food Ads Help Promote Bingeing or Binge Eating Disorders?

Pioneering activist, author, and ad critic Jean Kilbourne, EdD, has been sounding the alarm about junk-food advertising for more than four decades. Many of these spots, she cautions, "eroticize food and normalize bingeing" to the point of making it socially acceptable.[21]

Food and body image-related advertisements are subconsciously harming our relationship with what we eat, warned Kilbourne, whose groundbreaking documentary, *Killing Us Softly* (now in its fourth revision), spotlighted women's images in the media.

Recent research buttresses this point of view. Food products that are "advertised contain greater amounts of addictive ingredients, which encourage binge eating, resulting in an unprecedented obesity epidemic," warned Debbie Danowki, PhD, a Sacred Heart University associate communications professor and lead researcher of the study, "Bet You Can't Eat Just One: Binge Eating Disorder Promotion in American Food Advertising."[22]

Ninety-five percent of the ads reviewed by Dr. Danowski and her team included "representations of deep emotional attachment to food," and "87% of the ads included portrayals of [people] using food to replace relationships or as a way to bond with others," the researchers maintained in their study, which was published in *Media Literacy and Academic Research*.

The message conveyed was that "this food is special and eating it will provide great happiness, comfort and satisfaction," she continued.

The images shown in many food ads, Dr. Danowski asserted, "are designed to take away viewers' concerns about obesity and gaining weight from eating these products."

You're Forewarned and Forearmed

Now you have a flavor for some of the sophisticated, evocative, and emotionally manipulative ways Big Food (processed food companies) may use advertising, celebrity endorsements, or product placement to encourage you to eat their ultra-processed, sugary, fatty, salty food products.

Think back to when you overate. Did binge-watching or seeing ads with celebrities endorsing junk foods pave the way for you to eat badly, especially late at night? If so, place a check next to Reason #2 on your 21 Reasons I Blew My Diet List.

From now on, no matter what influencers or ads suggest, think for yourself. Just because certain singers, athletes, or stars appear in ad spots for sugary, fatty, salty junk foods or drinks doesn't mean you should take their dubious advice.

Instead, make your own buying decisions. Then take pride in the fact that you're stronger than those pervasive cues.

Beyond-the-Book Support: Make a Doctor's Appointment

While you learn 21 Reasons You Blew Your Diet, make an appointment for a medical checkup. Tell your health care provider that you're starting a plan to drop weight with the Bounce Back Diet. To find a doctor, go to my blog post at <u>www.connieb.com/ where-to-find-a-nutrition-savvy-doctor</u>.

Chapter 7

Why you blew your diet

You Craved and Overate Ultra-Processed Sweets and *Carbage* Designed to Hook You

What I found, over four years of research and reporting, was a conscious effort—taking place in labs and marketing meetings and grocery-store aisles—to get people hooked on [ultra-processed] foods that are convenient and inexpensive.[1]

—**Michael Moss**, Pulitzer Prize-winning journalist and author of the *New York Times* bestselling books *Salt Sugar Fat: How the Food Giants Hooked Us* and *Hooked: Food, Free Will, and How the Food Giants Exploit Our Addictions*

If you regularly overeat highly processed cookies, chips, or crackers, you may often wonder: "Why can't I ever get enough once I start?"

42

Don't blame yourself. Those refined concoctions are formulated to make you want to keep eating more and more and more.

The foods you crave are "knowingly designed—*engineered* is the better word—to maximize their allure," contends Michael Moss, author of *Salt Sugar Fat* and *Hooked*.[2]

For starters, major food manufacturers hired chemists who found ways to manipulate sugar, fat, and salt in processed foods to "purposely make them addictive," reveals Moss, a former *New York Times* reporter, who interviewed hundreds of food-industry insiders, inventors, and CEOs to explore why consumers keep coming back for more.[3]

Eye-Opening Food Industry Terms

Processed food manufacturers create refined, edible products to boost their *bottom lines*. But their financial goals can spell bad news for your *waistline*. The following industry terms offer some insights:

BLISS POINT

The *bliss point* is when the optimum amount of salt, sugar, or fat is added to processed foods to make their products so irresistible that they "send us over the moon" and "fly off the shelves," Moss explains.[4] The term was coined by market researcher and experimental psychologist Howard Moskowitz, PhD, in the 1950s.[5]

CRAVEABILITY, MOREISHNESS, SNACKABILITY

The terms need no explanations. Just know that food companies have devised ways to get you to eat as much as possible of their highly processed food concoctions.[6]

HEAVY USERS

These are the most loyal customers to whom the food industry targets the bulk of its marketing efforts. About 20 percent of consumers account for nearly 80 percent of the sales revenue.[7]

Why You Can't Stop: Highly Processed Carbs and Sweets "Bewitch" You

Wonder why it's so hard to stop eating extensively processed foods? They "bewitch" our taste buds into "a constant state of craving," Moss explains. [8]

One way food companies entice you to keep consuming highly processed sugary snacks and carbage is by adding sweeteners such as high fructose corn syrup, sucrose, and glucose.

The most addictive packaged foods are, in fact, those with added sugars, other sweeteners, or carbs. So found a study in *Nutrients* that looked at more than 230,000 processed food items sold in grocery stores, convenience stores, and fast-food outlets.[9] Companies even add sweeteners to foods not considered "sweet" such as crackers, breads, soup, mayonnaise, peanut butter, and tomato sauce.[10]

Sugar isn't the only driver of cravings. Research also shows that a fat-and-carb combo in a meal stimulates greater cravings, making it "supra-addictive."[11]

CARB SHOCKER!
Ultra-Processed Foods Make You Eat More

To understand how processed foods react differently in your body, let me tell you about a small but fascinating study published in *Cell Metabolism*. Twenty in-patients at the National Institutes of Health Clinical Center were assigned to eat two different diets. For the first two weeks, participants ate an ultra-processed menu. Then they switched to an unprocessed diet for the next fourteen days.

Both diets contained *almost identical* amounts of protein, carbs, fat, sugar, and salt. The only difference was *the degree to which the foods had been processed*. Those who ate ultra-processed foods took in about 500 more calories a day and gained nearly two pounds in two weeks. The takeaway? You'll eat more when you consume ultra-processed foods.[12]

Can Sweets and Highly Processed Carbs Be Addictive?

Let me reassure you if you feel frustrated by your consistent "need" for sweets or fast carbs. Over the years, mounting scientific research has explored whether people (or rats) can get over-attached to sweets or processed food substances.

Back in 2007, scientist Serge Ahmed, PhD, and his colleagues posed a pivotal question in the groundbreaking study, "Intense Sweetness Surpasses Cocaine Reward," which was published in *PLOS One*.[13]

"Our findings clearly demonstrate that intense sweetness can surpass cocaine reward, even in drug-sensitized and addicted individuals," concluded Dr. Ahmed, who heads addiction research at the French National Centre for Scientific Research at the University of Bordeaux in France.

Sugar acts on the reward center to encourage subsequent intake …
Whether it fits the criterion for addiction is irrelevant;
the stuff is abused.

—Robert H. Lustig, MD, pediatric endocrinologist;
YouTube sensation for his viral lecture, "Sugar: The Bitter Truth";
and *New York Times* bestselling author of *Fat Chance: Beating the Odds Against Sugar, Processed Food, Obesity, and Disease*

In recent years, other studies have explored similarities between sugar or carb addiction and drug addiction. Consider:

- **Highly processed foods were found to hijack your brain's reward centers.** Scientists found "strong evidence of the existence of sugar addiction," they stated in a review in *Frontiers in Psychiatry*.[15] The researchers discovered that both sugary foods and drugs release dopamine, the so-called pleasure hormone. The scholars suggested that "highly processed 'hyperpalatable' foods have hijacked the reward centers in the brain thus impairing the decision-making process, similar to drugs of abuse."[16] Sugar addiction, they found, also meets five of the eleven criteria for Substance Use Disorder (SUD), including the "use of larger amounts and for longer than intended, craving, hazardous use, tolerance, and withdrawal."

- **Processed foods share traits with other addictive substances.** For a study published in *PLOS One* and funded by the US government's National Institute on Drug Abuse (NIDA), other researchers speculated that highly processed foods are more likely to be associated with "addictive-like eating behaviors."[17]
- **Processed carbohydrates are the most addictive of all.** Neuroscientist Nicole Avena, PhD, observed that "it is not just the quantity of refined carbohydrates (like white flour and sugar) in a food, but the rapid speed in which they are absorbed into the system that is the most significant predictor of whether a particular food is associated with behavioral indicators of addictive-like eating."[18]

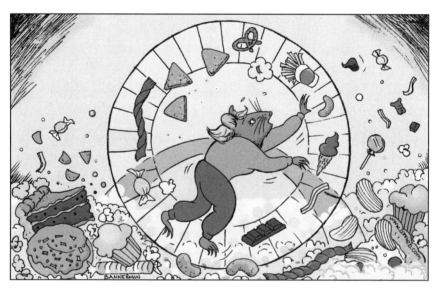

It's time to get off the sugar-addicted hamster wheel!

SUGAR SHOCKER!

Heroin is nothing but a chemical. They take the juice of the poppy and they refine it into opium and then they refine it to morphine and finally to heroin.

Sugar is nothing but a chemical. They take the juice of the cane or the beet and then refine it to molasses and then they refine it to brown sugar and finally to strange white crystals.[19]

—**William Dufty** (1916–2002), presenting the sugar-is-like-drugs argument in his 1975 bestseller *Sugar Blues*

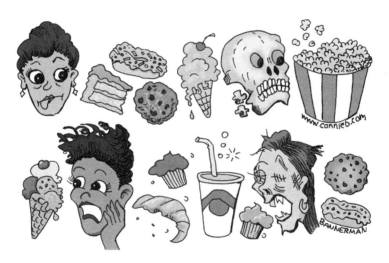

Scary! Your addictive carb or sugar habit may lead to diseases and even your untimely demise.

Are You a Sugar or Carb Addict?

What about you? Do you feel addicted to sugar and/or carbage? If the answer's yes, check off Reason #3 on your 21 Reasons List.

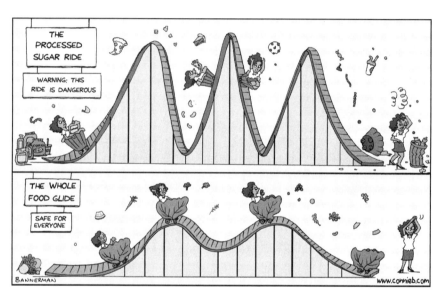

Are you stuck on the Blood Sugar Rollercoaster?

To see Isabella Bannerman's clever illustrations in color,
please visit my website, www.connieb.com, and click on the CARTOONS tab.

Chapter 8

REASON #4

Why you blew your diet

You Did *Blood Sugar* *Rollercoaster Scarfing*

If you're eating sugar throughout the day, you're spiking your blood sugar levels[s], and you're becoming a fat storing machine.[1]

—Jackie Warner, celebrity fitness trainer, TV personality, and *New York Times* bestselling author of *This Is Why You're Fat (And How to Get Thin Forever)*

Do you ever get so hungry that you feel like you could "eat a horse"?[2] Of course, this expression is absurd, but it conveys how people feel when they're in the middle of a low blood sugar reaction.

Let's see how this can play out on a typical day. Think back to a time you skipped breakfast or lunch or waited too long between meals while you were checking off items on your to-do list. Did you become fuzzy-headed, *hangry* (you know, hungry and angry), dizzy, shaky, and desperate for a candy bar? That's reactive hypoglycemia, or low blood sugar.

Most likely, at that point, in your frantic need for food to raise your blood sugar levels fast, you ignored your good intentions to eat healthier foods. You felt so crazy-hungry and out of sorts that you overate whatever foods were handy, especially sugary, fatty, salty processed snacks.[3]

> *The most fattening foods are the ones that have*
> *the greatest effect on our blood sugar and insulin levels.*[4]

—**Gary Taubes**, science journalist and the *New York Times* bestselling author of *Why We Get Fat* and *The Case Against Sugar*

How the Blood Sugar Rollercoaster Leads to Weight Gain

Unstable blood sugar levels are the archenemy of weight loss. When you eat sugar-filled desserts and fast carbs or drink sweetened beverages, you flood your bloodstream with sugar, also known as glucose.

Almost immediately, your blood sugar levels spike. This makes your pancreas release insulin, the hormone that ferries glucose from your bloodstream into cells where it's used as energy. That's why after eating a sweet snack, you feel a "sugar high."[5]

Glucose is the main source of fuel for your cells, especially your brain. In fact, you need glucose to stay alive. An optimal amount of glucose keeps your body humming, but too much wreaks havoc.

When you dump huge amounts of glucose into your body by eating processed carbs or sweet snacks, your pancreas jumps into overdrive to secrete more insulin to grab sugar out of your bloodstream and whisk it into your cells.[6]

The more glucose you pump into your bloodstream, the harder your pancreas needs to work. All that insulin transports excess glucose into your cells so quickly that you go from dangerously high blood sugar levels to crushingly low ones.

When your blood sugar levels crash some two to four hours later, you may become sluggish, irritable, headachy, dizzy, and famished. That's when you crave another sugar or carb "fix" to bring up your blood sugar levels.

Every few hours, you ride on the Blood Sugar Rollercoaster. Spike. Crash. Binge. And so on.

What happens to all that excess glucose in your bloodstream? It's stored in your liver to be used later as energy. When your liver runs out of room, extra glucose is stored as fat.[7]

How the Blood Sugar Rollercoaster Can Pack on Pounds

The research is irrefutable. Frequent blood sugar swings can lead to weight gain:

- **BMI increases as blood sugar levels soar, but the reverse is true, too.** For a study in the *Journal of Obesity and Chronic Diseases*, scientists measured the blood sugar levels and BMI of over 700 adults. They found that as blood sugar levels increased, so did BMI. On the other hand, balanced blood sugar levels helped the subjects shed weight. The researchers also discovered that the more physically active you are, the more protected you are from the association between elevated blood glucose and a higher BMI.[8]

- **A high-sugar diet can sour your moods.** After reviewing more than 300 studies, scientists writing in *Neuroscience & Biobehavioral Reviews* noticed that eating too many sweets can lead to anxiety, depression, and an increased impulse to overeat the same sugary junk foods that made participants feel bad in the first place.[9]

Blood Sugar Rollercoaster Scarfing

When you don't eat for two to four hours or longer, you may get dizzy, scattered, and hangry, because your blood sugar levels are so low. That's when you turn to processed carbs, sugary snacks, or drinks and do Blood Sugar Rollercoaster Scarfing. If you're like many Americans, you've been on this Blood Sugar Rollercoaster for years. Every day, you're spiking, crashing, and scarfing. What happens over time? Weight gain.

The Blood Sugar Rollercoaster
May Lead to Type 2 Diabetes

Weight gain isn't the only consequence of riding on the Blood Sugar Rollercoaster. Frequent blood sugar highs and lows can lead to a host of health problems.

"Hypoglycemia can be an important indicator of many chronic metabolic disorders," explains integrative physician Keith Berkowitz, MD, who considers reactive hypoglycemia "the Forgotten Blood Sugar Disorder."[10]

Many people wrongly believe that if you have reactive hypoglycemia and your blood sugar drops very low, you should suck hard candies or take a swig of orange juice, as do people with type 2 diabetes.

"If you have reactive hypoglycemia, the last thing you want to do is eat sugar," explains Dr. Berkowitz, medical director for the Center for Balanced Health in New York City. "With non-diabetic hypoglycemia, you want to bring up your blood sugar levels *more slowly* with healthy foods like almonds, a sugar-free protein shake, or a hard-boiled egg."[11]

If you think you may be going crazy; if you have thoughts of suicide; if you're constantly exhausted, anxious and depressed; if you go weeks without a decent night's sleep; if your personality changes like the flip of a coin; if a counter full of munchies doesn't satisfy your sweet tooth; and if your doctor thinks you must be a hypochondriac, because medical tests don't show anything physically wrong with you—don't despair, there's hope!

You may not need a psychiatrist, or even pain pills, tranquilizers or anti-depressants. Surprisingly, a simple DIET may relieve your symptoms!

This condition, which is confusing, complicated, misunderstood and too often misdiagnosed, is hypoglycemia, or low blood sugar.[12]

—**Roberta Ruggiero**, president and founder of the Hypoglycemia Support Foundation and author of *The Do's and Don'ts of Hypoglycemia: An Everyday Guide to Low Blood Sugar*

A growing number of physicians and metabolic experts now speculate that chronic low blood sugar (caused by a diet high in ultra-processed carbs and sweets) may be a precursor to type 2 diabetes.

The Hypoglycemia Support Foundation (HSF) explored this hypothesis by surveying 2,200 people with low blood sugar, many of whom went on to develop type 2 diabetes.[13] Most respondents with type 2 diabetes (68 percent) had symptoms of hypoglycemia before they received their diagnosis of type 2 diabetes.[14]

Meet the Real Carbs and Unreal Carbs

Not all carbs are bad for you. We need glucose from unprocessed, nutrient-dense carbs to fuel our brain and bodies, but some carbs are better for you than others. Let's review the differences:

Real Carbs or Best Carbs. These are the best, top quality, low glycemic carbs. They include superior, nonstarchy, low-carb vegetables such as asparagus, broccoli, cabbage, celery, cauliflower, cucumber, green beans, mushrooms, and zucchini. These veggies are made of long chains of glucose or sugar molecules, which means that they take a long time to digest and don't spike your blood sugar levels.[15]

Naturally Occurring Simple Carbs. Don't be fooled by the word "natural." Carbs from high-sugar fruits, white potatoes, fruit juices, and smoothies cause huge blood sugar spikes. You also want to be wary of high-sugar fruits such as watermelon, bananas, raisins, dates, and mangoes.[16]

Unreal Carbs. These inferior carbs have been stripped of their fiber and nutritional value with high-powered machinery.[17] These carbs are high glycemic, which means that they quickly dump glucose into your bloodstream and cause an immediate jump in your blood sugar levels. Unreal carbs include white rice, white breads, gluten flours, fruit juice, most cookies, crackers, candies, and chips, as well as caloric sweeteners such as table sugar, barley malt, coconut sugar, and evaporated cane juice.

To conclude, loading up on Unreal Carbs can lead to weight gain, blood sugar issues, and addiction. On the other hand, consuming healthy, quality, low-glycemic Real Carbs or Best Carbs can, along with ample protein and fat, make you feel better and facilitate weight loss.

For many people, eating involves constant swings from unpleasantly hungry to uncomfortably full. On this roller-coaster ride, highly processed food may provide a few minutes of enjoyment, but it quickly sets us up for the next downward swing, with negative effects on our physical and mental well-being.[18]

—**David Ludwig, MD, PhD**, endocrinologist, researcher at Boston Children's Hospital, Harvard School of Public Health nutrition professor, and author of *Always Hungry?: Conquer Cravings, Retrain Your Fat Cells, and Lose Weight Permanently*

A Primer on Blood Sugar Conditions

Research reveals that either well-managed or poorly controlled blood sugar levels can affect your short- and long-term health, including your body's ability to maintain healthy weight. These are the blood sugar imbalances:

Hypoglycemia, reactive (or low blood sugar). This is usually caused by consuming large amounts of high-glycemic carbs and refined sugars. You've already learned that within two to four hours of eating these foods, your blood sugar levels may plummet below the normal range. Common low blood sugar symptoms include headaches, dizziness, confusion, depression, and sugar or carb cravings.[19]

Insulin resistance. When you overeat sugar or processed carbs that quickly break down into glucose, your pancreas needs to produce more insulin. Over time, your cells begin to adjust to these new, higher levels, and your body requires more insulin to transport glucose to the cells until the pancreas stops responding. This is called insulin resistance.[20]

Metabolic syndrome. This is a group of related conditions that afflicts one in three American adults and raises your risk for stroke, type 2 diabetes, and heart disease. High blood sugar can contribute to metabolic syndrome, because it puts stress on blood vessels.[21]

Prediabetes. When your blood sugar levels are chronically elevated but aren't high enough to be diagnosed as type 2 diabetes, you may have prediabetes. This condition increases the risk of developing type 2 diabetes, heart disease, and stroke. An estimated 96 million American adults have prediabetes, and more than eight in ten people don't know they have it.[22]

Type 1 diabetes. Once known as juvenile diabetes or insulin-resistant diabetes, this autoimmune disease is usually diagnosed early and believed to be inherited. With type 1 diabetes, the pancreas doesn't release any insulin so patients need to inject synthetic insulin every day. Type 1 diabetes affects nearly 1.9 million Americans.[23]

Type 2 diabetes. This disease comprises up to 95 percent of all cases of diabetes. It can be caused by extra weight around the mid-section, as well as such unhealthy lifestyle habits as a poor diet and lack of physical activity. Approximately 33 million to 35 million Americans have type 2 diabetes.[24]

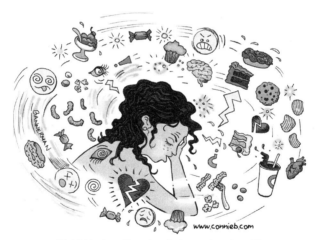

"Ugh! I feel so dizzy, headachy, and confused!"

Blood Sugar Issues Are Rampant Today

So how many people in the United States regularly ride on the Blood Sugar Rollercoaster? A study published in *JAMA* suggested that nearly 50 percent of adults have diabetes or prediabetes.[25]

What about you? Have you been doing Blood Sugar Rollercoaster Scarfing? If so, check Reason #4 on your 21 Reasons List.

Hang tight, because this book helps you get off that dangerous ride.

Chapter 9

Why you blew your diet

Heartbreak Bingeing Hurried in after a Loved One Died

After the death of my dad and my divorce, I was devastated. I felt a massive hole in my heart so I plugged the hole with sugar. Lots of it. Within six months, I gained 15 pounds. But the sugar was making me feel worse. My lethargy, headaches, racing heart and disturbed sleep were just awful.[1]

—**Theresa**, 54

We now need to look at the toughest transition we will all face at some point in our lives—the death of someone dear to us.

The loss of a beloved mother, father, husband, wife, partner, parental figure, child, or baby is so incredibly painful that it can trigger a ramped-up, frantic, no-holds-barred overeating that I call *Heartbreak Bingeing*.

If this hits home, let me share my deep condolences for your loss—no matter when it happened. My heart goes out to you.

Before we explore how losing a loved one may pave the way for you to binge on junk foods and pack on pounds, let's take another quick mental health break.

We'll do the simple Breathe, Yawn, Play Process you practiced earlier.[2] To refresh your memory, just take three slow, deep breaths. Next, mindfully yawn three times. Then play the soothing composition "Weightless" from Marconi Union.[3]

How I Discovered the Grieving and Bingeing Connection

As I shared in Chapter 1, my eating quickly spun out of control after a grueling year helplessly watching a terminal cancer end my mother's life. Determined to take charge of my eating and get out of my funk, I attended numerous self-help events and workshops where I met other grief-stricken people.

It was uncanny how alike our experiences were. Someone special died. We felt devastated. We overate. We gained weight. We felt ashamed. We longed to heal after our losses, drop our excess weight, and reclaim our power.

As both a grieving overeater and curious journalist, I felt driven to investigate. Turns out I was onto a phenomenon. The Germans have a word for "the weight a person gains during a period of overeating due to unhappiness, depression, grief, or other emotional condition," according to Dictionary.com. They call the extra pounds *kummerspeck*, which translates to "grief bacon," "sad fat," "worry weight," or "sorrow flab."[4]

In my case, I was startled by the intensity, fervor, and speed with which I pigged out after my loss. Never had I done this kind of frenzied gorging. Other mourners shared eerily similar stories. After delving into this phenomenon, it became clear to me that while deep in our sorrow, we'd been doing Heartbreak Bingeing.

Heartbreak Bingeing

When you're reeling from a broken heart over the death of a loved one, you may do a type of frantic, frenetic, furious overeating that I call Heartbreak Bingeing. You're so overcome by overpowering emotional pain that you quickly stuff down enormous amounts of junk foods. Like other ways of overeating, Heartbreak Bingeing may last for weeks, months, or years and lead to rapid weight gain and poorer health. This is one of what I call the *Big Four Binge Triggers*.

Heartbreak Bingeing Is One of the Most Dangerous Types of Overeating

You've no doubt heard of the term "emotional eating." That phrase doesn't come anywhere close to describing the kind of gorging I'm discussing. Heartbreak Bingeing takes escaping into food to a whole new level. Your eating is desperate, drastic, dangerous.

When your eating is fueled by gut-wrenching despair, complicated grief, and many woulda-coulda-shoulda thoughts, you can demolish massive amounts of junk foods and hundreds, if not thousands, of calories in mere minutes. Within weeks or months, you're likely busting out of your clothes.

Of course, Heartbreak Bingeing never helps you escape your grief. In the aftermath, things get worse. You feel more depressed, hopeless, and down on yourself.

On top of that, Heartbreak Bingeing can jeopardize your health because you packed on so many pounds. Ultimately, this serious type of overeating can wreak havoc on all aspects of your being—physical, emotional, and spiritual.

After spending more than seven years researching why people blew their diets, I've come to believe that the death of a favorite person (especially a mother, father, husband, wife, child, or baby) is such an incredibly painful life change that I classify it as one of the *Big Four Binge Triggers*. The other three overeating activators are a breakup or divorce, trauma, and caregiving, which we'll discuss in the next three chapters.

> *In the face of loss, I gained. Time passed,*
> *someone else died, and my body grew, becoming a*
> *visible archive of each late-night ice cream binge,*
> *every delivery order snuck past my roommates so*
> *I could eat ashamedly and privately in my bedroom.*[5]

—**Jehan Roberson**, "I Ate My Way Through Grief:
How four deaths in 18 months changed my
body," published on www.Vice.com

Grief Can Alter Your Appetite

Of course, everyone grieves differently after a loved one dies.

"There is no 'normal' appetite in grief," observes grief expert and psychotherapist Megan Devine, LPC, author of *It's OK That You're Not OK: Meeting Grief and Loss in a Culture That Doesn't Understand.*[6] "Some people eat under stress; some people lose all interest in food."

But lack of appetite doesn't last long. "After a major loss such as the death of a loved spouse or partner, the appetite for food is often the first appetite to return," British psychiatrist and grief expert Colin Murray Parkes, MD, explained in an article in the *BMJ*. By the third or fourth month of grieving, he discovered, the lost weight is "found."[7]

Then about the sixth month after the loss, "many people have put on too much weight," Dr. Parkes observed. "It may be many more months before people begin to care about their appearances, and for sexual and social appetites to return."

> *Grief has just turned me into*
> *a lazy lump of dough.*[8]

—**Participant** in a Reddit forum

Of Grieving, Bingeing, and Weight Gain

Let's now explore some eye-opening research that connects the death of a loved one with overeating:

- **Grieving may lead to binge eating.** One study looked at more than 5,100 people and found an association between the death of a family member and a higher BMI between four to eight years after the loss. Bereavement may "lead to binge eating and poor eating habits that serve to help a survivor dull his/her senses, relieve sorrow and escape emotional pain, which may lead to an increase in BMI," concluded the study, which was published in *PLOS One*.[9] Grieving people "may use food as 'self-medication' because sweet tastes have mood-elevating and pain-suppressing properties." Interestingly, when it came to losing a mother or father, both women and men were hit hard.

- **After losing a spouse, the remaining partner may consume more comfort foods.** A study in *Comprehensive Psychoneuroendocrinology* found that for at least two years after the death of a spouse, the loss significantly increased the likelihood of eating highly saturated fatty snacks and comfort foods.[10]

- **Stressful life events, such as the death of a loved one, may trigger binge-eating disorder.** A study in *Psychiatry Research* found that people who suffer from binge-eating disorder (BED) are more likely to be triggered by stressful life events, including the death of a loved one. The researchers suggested that grief and bereavement triggered BED in these subjects.[11]

- **Adverse life experiences may lead to obesity and BED.** After reviewing seventy studies that looked at nearly 307,000 participants, researchers writing in the *Journal of Behavioral Addictions* observed a strong association (87 percent) between adverse life experiences, obesity, and BED.[12]

After my step dad passed away, I gained 70 pounds in 3 months. I didn't like how I felt or looked… [I]t's so important for me to look back and tell that man from 5 years ago he was lovely… I can celebrate where I am now as long as I send love to the 'me's' along the way.[13]

—**Jonathan Van Ness,** hair stylist and grooming advisor for the reality show *Queer Eye*

Love Yourself and Honor Your Beloved

Am I talking about your situation? Have you been doing Heartbreak Bingeing after the death of a loved one? If so, mark a check next to Reason #5 on your 21 Reasons List.

Now, if you're still grieving the loss of someone special to you, it's important to get support. "What we run from pursues us. What we face transforms us," explains grief expert David Kessler, author of *Finding Meaning: The Sixth Stage of Grief.*

You want to make "a decision [to move through grief]," advises Kessler, also the coauthor with Louise Hay of *You Can Heal Your Heart.*[14]

"The meaning is what we do after the loss," Kessler amplifies.

"Do we just go through our grief, or do we grow through it?"[15]

While you face your grief, this is also a good time to do activities in honor of the person you lost.

Listen to her favorite music. Donate to his favorite charity. Take a walk in her favorite park. Then, live with gusto.

Isn't that what your loved one would want?

Beyond-the-Book Support:
Where to Get Grief Support

If you're mourning the loss of a loved one, you'll find a list of helpful resources to set you on a path to healing at www.connieb.com/where-to-get-grief-support.

Chapter 10

REASON #6

Why you blew your diet

Breaking Up Is Hard
. . . On Your Diet

*After my divorce, food became my fun, my release, my drug of
choice. I definitely self-medicated. . . . There was nobody there to
stop me or be disgusted by how much I was ingesting.*

*I gained 20 pounds from the time I knew I was getting a divorce to
the time I moved out. The food was comforting until I didn't feel good
about myself anymore. I felt swollen and blown up with extra weight,
and I couldn't fit into my clothes. I was in a vicious cycle.[1]*

—**Jamie D.**, 44, Pennsylvania

Tina Turner's hit song "What's Love Got to Do with It?" kept playing
in my mind while I was writing this chapter.[2] That's because love

can have an awful lot to do with your weight. Indeed, relationships on the rocks or on the outs account for another of the Big Four Binge Triggers. There are three ways a stormy or fading relationship with your spouse, ex, or live-in partner could play a big role in why you ate badly and packed on pounds.

Types of Overeating Triggered by Relationships on the Rocks

BICKERING BINGEING. If you're angry at your honey, you may thoughtlessly reach for unhealthy what-nots rather than calmly chat to clear the air. Enter Bickering Bingeing.

BREAKUP BINGEING. You and your sweetie called it quits. Now you may be vainly trying to fill the void and deal with your heartbreak by turning to processed sweets and carb comfort foods. That's Breakup Bingeing.

DIVORCE DEVOURING. Your partner has moved out, made plans to leave, or you're about to sign divorce papers. During this upsetting transition and afterwards, your eating may escalate to Divorce Devouring.

The Unhappy-Together-or-Apart Bingeing Effect

In looking at how troubled relationships can lead to growing girth, I discovered some startling studies. For instance:

- **People whose marriages are on the rocks may gain weight.** After monitoring the BMIs of nearly 9,500 people for more than a decade, researchers writing in the *American Journal of Public Health* concluded that if a marriage was troubled, both partners gained weight. Couples who experienced stress in their relationships were more likely than happier couples to add a couple of inches to their waistlines and experience an increase in BMI of 10 percent or more.[3]

- **Stress in troubled marriages can lead to bigger tummies.** Married women and men added an average of 10 percent to their weight or four inches to their waist over four years when they were anxious about their relationship, suggested scholars who followed more than 2,000 married couples who were together an average of 34 years. "The stress experienced by partners, and not the individual's stress, was associated with increased waist circumference," observed Kira Birditt, PhD, lead author of the study that was published in *The Journals of Gerontology.*[4]

- **Divorced people may pack on pounds.** After examining data on nearly 20,950 men and women over sixteen years, investigators discovered that "relationship transitions" may lead to an increase in BMI. "Divorce generally predicted weight gain," suggested the study published in *Health Psychology.*[5]

Children of Parents in Troubled Marriages May Gain Weight, Too

Research shows that when a couple separates or divorces, the unhappy home life may lead the children to gain weight. After analyzing data on more than 7,500 children, investigators found that kids whose parents separated were significantly more likely to become overweight or obese within three years of the split. The study, published in the journal *Demography*, discovered that weight gain was most pronounced in children whose parents separated when the kids were age six or younger.[6]

Forget Getting a "Revenge Body" —Go for a Healthier Body

We can't discuss the connection between splitting up and weight without addressing the controversial concept of getting a "revenge body."[7] That's when a person may seek to lose weight and tone up to show a former spouse, same-sex partner, boyfriend, or girlfriend that she or he is doing just fine, thank you, without the ex.

The idea of getting a revenge body misses the point. You want a healthier body *for you*, not a kick-ass body to impress or spite your ex. Instead, I recommend that you get "revenge" in better ways.

Use this time after a breakup to make health a top priority. Banish your junky thoughts. Snub junk foods that got you hooked. Decide that your *breakup* will lead to a *breakthrough*.

You know what comes next. Decide if Reason #6 holds true for you.

Have you been doing Bickering Bingeing, Breakup Bingeing, or Divorce Devouring? If so, check which type applies to you on your 21 Reasons List.

Beyond-the-Book Support: Types of Overeating

Overeating can be alarming, embarrassing, and dangerous. To discover the types of bingeing or disordered eating that I discuss in this book, get your gift at www.BounceBackDiet.com/Book-Bonuses.

Chapter 11

Why you blew your diet

You Relied on *Comfort Crunching* While Reeling from Trauma

All of us who have been broken and scarred by trauma have the chance to turn those experiences into . . . post-traumatic wisdom.

Because what I know for sure is that everything that has happened to you was also happening for you. And all that time, in all of those moments, you were building strength.

Strength times strength times strength equals power. What happened to you can be your power.[1]

—Oprah Winfrey, from the *New York Times* bestseller, *What Happened to You?: Conversations on Trauma, Resilience, and Healing*, with psychiatrist and neuroscientist **Bruce D. Perry, MD, PhD**

Trauma.
Do a Google search for the word, and you get nearly 1.9 *billion* hits.[2] Clearly, something is greatly amiss.

People are yearning for help to deal with stressful, frightening, or life-threatening events that adversely impacted their lives.

Let's jump right to the eating connection. An unthinkable or horrifying incident you witnessed or experienced—even if it happened years ago—may be why you've been bingeing on junk foods.

Before we inspect this sensitive subject, let's take another Breathe, Yawn, Play time out. Remember, take three slow, deep, calming breaths; mindfully yawn three times; and listen to Marconi Union's "Weightless."[3]

> *Trauma is perhaps the most avoided, ignored, belittled,*
> *denied, misunderstood, and untreated cause of human suffering.*[4]
>
> —**Peter A. Levine, PhD**, psychotherapist and
> author of *Waking the Tiger: Healing Trauma*

How Does PTSD Develop?

Before I delve into the binge-eating connection, let me share a little history. Trauma is nothing new. It's been "part of the human condition since we evolved as a species," according to the National Center for PTSD, a division of the US Department of Veterans Affairs.[5]

For centuries, soldiers returning from battle or survivors of wars experienced what was called "shell shock," "combat fatigue," "war neurosis," "railroad spine," or "soldier's heart."[6] Finally, in the 1970s, people became increasingly aware of trauma's far-reaching effects when one-third of Vietnam War veterans suffered from depression, episodic combat flashbacks, and drug or alcohol problems.[7]

But trauma isn't limited to veterans. In fact, 70 percent of US adults—or more than 223 million people—have experienced a traumatic event at least once in their lives, according to the National Council for Mental Wellbeing.[8]

After going through a traumatic incident, people may develop post-traumatic stress disorder, or PTSD. This mental health condition can occur after surviving gun violence, a natural disaster, serious accident, terrorist attack, rape or sexual assault, intimate partner violence, serious injury, or the unexpected death of a loved one. PTSD also can stem from bullying, childhood abuse or neglect, cultural or intergenerational trauma, emotional exploitation, disloyalty, infidelity, or backstabbing.[9]

PTSD knows no bounds. It can occur in "all people, of any ethnicity, nationality or culture, and at any age," according to the American Psychiatric Association.[10]

Interestingly, although males have a greater chance of experiencing traumatic events, females are twice as likely to get PTSD, according to the American Psychological Association.[11]

So how do you know if you, a loved one, or colleague has PTSD?

Here are some telltale signs: long after the traumatic event ended, the person may become hypervigilant, easily startled or frightened; feel sad, depressed, irritable, anxious, angry, become emotionally numb, experience flashbacks and nightmares, find it tough to concentrate, have trouble falling or staying asleep, be socially isolated, and avoid people, places, or things that trigger reminders of the traumatizing event(s).[12]

In addition, someone who has PTSD may engage in self-destructive behavior such as drinking too much or overeating.[13] Naturally, our focus in this book is how your bingeing or altered eating may have started, escalated, or worsened after you experienced trauma.

Trauma is not the bad things that happened to you, but what happens inside you as a result of what happened to you.[14]

—**Gabor Maté**, **MD**, expert on addiction, trauma, and stress
and *New York Times* bestselling author, with Daniel Maté,
of *The Myth of Normal: Trauma, Illness, and Healing in a Toxic Culture*

Trauma Awareness Has Surged in Recent Years

In the past decade, trauma has risen to the forefront of our consciousness, thanks, in large part, to the widely popular book *The Body Keeps the Score: Brain, Mind, and Body in the Healing of Trauma* by psychiatrist, educator, and trauma researcher Bessel Van der Kolk, MD.[15]

"Trauma affects the entire human organism—body, mind, and brain," he wrote in the 2014 book, which had spent 303 weeks on the *New York Times* bestseller list while I was completing this book.[16]

"In PTSD the body continues to defend against a threat that belongs to the past," Dr. Van der Kolk explains. "Healing from PTSD means being able to terminate this continued stress mobilization and restore the entire organism to safety."

"The big issue for traumatized people is that they don't own themselves anymore. Any loud sound, anybody insulting them, hurting them, saying bad things can hijack them away from themselves," Dr. Van der Kolk said in an interview. "And so what we have learned is that what makes you resilient to trauma is to own yourself fully."[17]

[Y]our past traumas are your "Sacred Wounds." Because wherever you have suffered the most is where you have the opportunity to contribute the most.[18]

—**Katherine Woodward Thomas**, licensed marriage and family therapist, author of *Calling in "The One"* and *Conscious Uncoupling*

How I Stumbled onto the Trauma-Binge Eating Connection

Up until a few years ago, all I knew about PTSD was that war veterans suffer from it. But after that painful year with my dying mom, in between doing lots of Heartbreak Bingeing, I was beset by such baffling symptoms as severe insomnia, flashbacks, and hypervigilance.

For instance, if a frisky dog suddenly barked near me, I jumped, screeched, and went on high alert. Talk about embarrassing! Because I was so alarmed by my strange reactions, I consulted two specialists, both of whom confirmed that my responses were indicative of PTSD.

While reviewing medical studies for this book, I finally connected the dots. My out-of-the-blue bingeing after losing Mom finally made sense. The brutal, stressful, heartbreaking year had triggered *both* PTSD and trauma-triggered overeating.

That important insight led me to identify and coin another type of bingeing that many traumatized grievers do. Meet *Comfort Crunching*.

Comfort Crunching

You've been traumatized and developed PTSD after one or more life-changing events, such as the death of a loved one, a natural disaster, sexual assault, gun violence, a terrorist attack, betrayal by a close family member, or intergenerational trauma.[19]

Even if the terrifying event occurred years ago, it may still be affecting you. You've been feeling so desperate, discouraged, or depressed that you've frantically gobbled candies, cookies, and other junk foods.

Comfort Crunching is especially dangerous, because it can lead to rapid weight gain and numerous health challenges. Experiencing trauma is one of the Big Four Binge Triggers.

Research That Connects Trauma to Binge Eating

If you, too, have been traumatized, *and* you've been binge-eating for months or years, you may have been doing Comfort Crunching. Research reveals that traumatic experiences, as well as childhood abuse, neglect, and betrayal, may increase a person's risk for obesity, binge eating disorder, bulimia, and anorexia nervosa. Check out some eye-opening studies that explore these connections:

- **Trauma may trigger bingeing.** A study in *The Journal of Clinical Psychiatry* that analyzed data from more than 36,300 adults surveyed by The National Epidemiologic Survey on Alcohol and Related Conditions found that people who developed binge-eating habits were more likely to have experienced high levels of trauma in their lives. "Much like drugs and alcohol, binge-eating is used as a strategy to deal with trauma," the scientists concluded.[20]
- **PTSD is connected to becoming overweight or obese.** A study in *JAMA Psychiatry* notes that "a growing body of evidence suggests that PTSD is an important risk factor for obesity and obesity-related diseases, including type 2 diabetes and cardiovascular disease." Spe-

cifically, the researchers found that women with one to three PTSD symptoms had an 18 percent risk of becoming overweight or obese, and ladies with at least four symptoms had a 36 percent greater chance of gaining weight. Those findings were based on responses from more than 50,500 females, who were a subsample of participants in the famous, large-scale, multiyear Nurses' Health Study II.[21]

- **Overeating after enduring trauma is common.** A study of more than 3,000 adult women that was published in the *Journal of Obesity & Eating Disorders* found that those who had been victims of crimes such as rape, attempted murder, and molestation were more likely to develop bulimia nervosa and PTSD compared to the general population. They also were far more likely to be obese.[22]
- **Sexual abuse may lead to disordered eating.** Researchers who looked at data on more than 12,000 survivors of sexual violence found that they had *nearly four times* the odds of developing disordered eating later in life compared to those without PTSD, scientists revealed in their study in *Eating and Weight Disorders*.[23] (Disordered eating refers to such irregular eating behaviors as compulsive eating, restrictive dieting, or skipping meals.)

Whoa! Are you as dumbfounded as I was when I first discovered the connection between trauma and binge eating, obesity, and/or eating disorders?

Take Heart! You Can Move on to a Great Life after Trauma

If you've been traumatized, let me offer you hope for a brighter future. Research shows that after difficult life events, survivors may ultimately develop an increased appreciation of life, take more pleasure in small things, have improved relationships, find greater personal strength, be more open to new possibilities, and become more spiritual. Experts call this *post-traumatic growth* (PTG).[24]

The wound is the place where the light enters you.[25]

—**Rumi**, 13th-century Persian poet

"People who've gone through shattering experiences . . . [can] use them as fuel for the transformational journey," contends scientist, health researcher, and EFT Universe founder Dawson Church, PhD.[26]

He should know. After narrowly escaping seconds before a California wildfire engulfed his home and office, developing a painful medical condition, and experiencing financial disaster, Dr. Church bounced back and even wrote the book *Bliss Brain: The Neuroscience of Remodeling Your Brain for Resilience, Creativity, and Joy.*

"We can use even the most devastating loss as a springboard for growth," he now insists.

Indeed, let me assure you that you can face and rise above your old ordeals. Although trauma threw you topsy-turvy, it needn't stomp out your spark. The sweet irony is that your trauma-triggered bingeing can now become a pathway to your power.

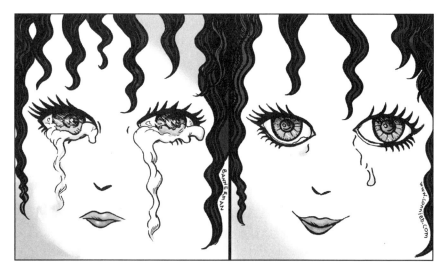

You, too, can heal after trauma and move from sad to glad.

Is Comfort Crunching Your Achilles Heel?

It's time to look dispassionately at your bingeing behavior. Have you been doing Comfort Crunching due to lingering PTSD? Go to your 21 Reasons list. Now check off Reason # 7 (Comfort Crunching) if that's why you've been eating badly.

Chapter 12

REASON #8

Why you blew your diet

Watching Your Loved One Suffer Set Off *Caregiving Chomping*

Caretaking itself does not cause weight gain,
but careless eating while caretaking does.[1]

—**Mary** (pseudonym), in an online forum on AgingCare.com

When her mother was suffering from dementia, Jeanne Erdmann was her primary caregiver. In particular, the last five years of her mom's life were "really tough, stressful, and exhausting," recalls Erdmann, who "grabbed more and more comfort foods such as cupcakes, French fries, and soft ice cream."[2]

"Even with small breaks, I could never get fully rested," adds Erdmann, a health and science journalist, who has written for *Discover*, the *Washington Post*, *Nature*, *Slate*, and many other outlets.

Every year, about one in five Americans or 53 million adults are caregivers like Erdmann. They provide unpaid care to a chronically ill or disabled family member with special needs, according to the National Alliance for Caregiving and the AARP.[3]

If you're a full or part-time caregiver, you deserve the utmost respect for taking on this important role.

While you pour your heart into watching over your loved one, you put in long hours and are often isolated while you witness the suffering or physical deterioration of your family member.[4]

Monitoring an ailing mother or father is one form of caregiving. You also may be a parent who does double duty. As part of the "sandwich generation," you care for your kid(s), with or without special needs or an illness, *and* one or both older parent(s).[5]

Caregiving can be unbelievably stressful and endlessly demanding while you juggle many duties, including managing medications, preparing meals, communicating with doctors, and providing companionship and emotional support, according to CaringInfo.org.[6]

Your unique situation makes you especially vulnerable to doing another kind of overeating. Meet Caregiving Chomping.

Caregiving Chomping

This is when the stress, strain, and tension of caring for your ailing or terminally-ill loved one or child, with or without special needs, drives you to nibble or binge on fast, easy, convenient junk foods. In between watching your kids or loved one succumb to a chronic disease or other health issues, you may ignore your needs. Caregiving Chomping is one of the Big Four Binge Triggers.

When You're a Caregiver, It's Easy to Skip Self-Care

Caregivers face a particular dilemma. When you're dedicated to watching your loved one, you may stop doing good-for-you activities. Consider:

- **Caregivers are in "poorer health than the rest of the nation."** Those taking care of others have "higher rates of high cholesterol, high blood pressure, overweight/obesity and depression," according to an American Psychological Association Stress in America survey. Caregivers also are "far more likely than the general population to lay awake at night" (60 percent vs. 44 percent).[7]
- **Depression and anxiety among caregivers are common.** Between 40 percent and 70 percent of caregivers show symptoms of either depression or anxiety, according to a review published in *Medicine*.[8]

> *To care for those who once cared for us*
> *is one of the highest honors.*[9]

—**Tia Walker,** author of *The Inspired Caregiver:*
Finding Joy While Caring for Those You Love

Overeating Is Common among Caregivers

Given the huge load on caregivers, stressed and depressed caregivers may turn to junk foods. For instance:

- **Caregivers may gain weight.** After looking at more than 12,000 caregivers and nearly 46,000 noncaregivers, those watching loved ones were more inclined to be sedentary. The caregivers also had a greater likelihood of being overweight or obese compared to noncaregivers, according to a study in the *International Journal of Public Health*.[10]
- **Caregivers may skip self-care.** About 63 percent of caregivers reported that their eating habits were worse than before, and 58 percent shared that they weren't exercising as much as they did before they took on caregiving responsibilities, according to a survey from the National Alliance of Caregiving and Evercare.[11]

- **Mothers with extra caring responsibilities may have bigger waists and increased diabetes risk.** Investigators looking at the eating habits of mothers with the stress of caring for autistic children were more likely to reward themselves with food. Nearly twice as many mothers with autistic children also met the criteria for significant insulin resistance, according to the study in *Family Process*.[12]

> *Give yourself credit for doing the best you can*
> *in one of the toughest jobs there is.*[13]
>
> **—Caregiver Action Network (CAN)**

You Need to Care for Yourself, Too

If you're a caregiver, it's small wonder that you feel exhausted, frustrated, and anxious. But this is no time to eat junk foods and be sedentary. You need to ramp up self-care. Your loved one needs you to be strong and healthy.

When you learn to manage stress better and are well nourished, you'll find it easier to have the patience, courage, and stamina to be a good caregiver.

Did I describe your situation? Are you watching a terminally ill parent or child with disability? Did that difficult situation lead you to do Caregiving Chomping? If that's the case, mark Reason #8 on your 21 Reasons List.

Chapter 13

REASON #9

Why you blew your diet

Trying Times Triggered Stress Splurging

Stressed spelled backwards is desserts. Coincidence? I think not![1]

—**Loretta LaRoche**, stress management consultant and humorist

When stress strikes, Lorena D. often feels "drawn to carbs."[2] But polishing off a big bag of chips or other junk foods "doesn't actually relieve the stress," she admits.

Lorena is like millions who've anxiously grabbed and gobbled nutrient-lacking sugary, salty, fatty processed comfort foods.

Let's face it, the United States is one stressed-out nation. Indeed, nearly two-thirds of American adults felt overwhelmed by a "barrage of external stressors," according to a Stress in America survey conducted by the Harris Poll for the American Psychological Association.[3]

No matter what your reasons for stress, it often leads to unhealthy habits, including less physical activity, worse sleep, higher rates of drinking alcohol, and eating more junk foods.

Stress Splurging

When you face a steady stream of stress, anxiety, and worry over a variety of issues, you're more likely to binge on carbage, sweet snacks, or fast foods. *Stress Splurging* is one of the most common, fattening, and harmful ways of overeating. During the first year of the Covid pandemic, while stress soared to unparalleled heights, millions of people did a type of Stress Splurging that I call *Pandemic Pigging Out.*

How Modern-Day Stress Accelerates

When you're feeling stress, your body releases a flood of *cortisol,* the "fight-or-flight" hormone linked to cravings for foods that provide quick energy, such as simple high-glycemic carbs and sweets.[4]

Back in prehistoric times, cortisol helped our ancestors escape from those voracious saber-toothed tigers. Cut to modern times. We're no longer running from such frightening creatures. Today, our stresses are more insidious and constant.

For instance, we may be stressed about our romantic relationships, children, parents, health issues, finances, inflation, work, global uncertainty, racial injustice, gun violence, political divisiveness, and climate change.

Of Stress, Sweets, Carbs, and Your Waistline

Over the years, studies have explored the connection between stress, elevated cortisol, and weight gain. For instance:

- **Stress-triggered cortisol leads to bigger waists.** A study in *Obesity* found that women who were obese had the most significant amounts of cortisol.[5]
- **People eat sugary foods and calories when they're under stress.** Researchers from the Institute of Psychiatry in London found that elevated levels of cortisol during a period of chronic stress were strongly correlated with a higher intake of calories, sugar, and saturated fat. That led to weight gain, scientists shared in the *European Eating Disorders Review*.[6]

> *At the beginning of quarantine, I definitely gained the quarantine 15. I was literally in the living room . . . looking at myself in the mirror [and thinking . . .] "Wow, girl you have really done it. 'Why are you baking so much? How many Honeybuns can we eat?"*
>
> *[Then I realized], "You look good though. We should dance about it.' . . . The ["body-ody"] hook literally came from me dancing in the mirror and admiring my fluff. [This] song [is] definitely about people just celebrating their bodies.[7]*
>
> —**Megan Thee Stallion**, rapper, singer, songwriter,
> talking about her hit song, "Body-ody" on
> *The Late Show with Stephen Colbert*

Stress Splurging Skyrocketed as Covid Spread

Perhaps the best example of Stress Splurging run wild occurred during the first year of the coronavirus pandemic in 2020, when millions were worried about getting the disease, concerned about the safety of their children and elderly relatives, and feeling increasingly isolated.

Covid and the resulting lockdowns led people to eat more junk foods, exercise less, become more anxious, and get less sleep, according to a study in *Obesity*.[8]

During that first year of Covid, two in five packed on more than fifteen pounds, according to the American Psychological Association's Pandemic Anniversary Survey conducted by the Harris Poll. The average weight increase was higher, about twenty-nine pounds.[9]

While I'm not at the weight I want to be, the reality is that loving your body ONLY when it's a "perfect shape" (whatever that is) is like only loving your kids when they are well-behaved. So, let's take a moment to appreciate the curves, shall we?[10]

—**Jennifer "Jay" Palumbo**, writer, stand-up comic, and mompreneur in a tweet on #plussizeappreciationday

Let's Accept Our Bodies No Matter What

As the world began to open up, many people had challenges fitting into their favorite prepandemic clothes.[11]

Journalist Virginia Sole-Smith, who writes about weight stigma, antifat bias, and diet culture, suggested that "when we get hit with that tidal wave of 'none of my pants fit!' instead of dieting, we can start by asking ourselves what we're really worrying about, underneath or alongside the pants thing.[12]

"Let's name that fear or worry (or multiple fears and worries) rather than letting it silently fester," urged Sole-Smith, author of *Fat Talk: Parenting in the Age of Diet Culture.*

Remember, she insisted, that "we are always allowed to be imperfect."

When many people gained weight during Covid, the body positivity movement gathered momentum.[13] The term "body positive" was coined in 1996 when psychotherapist Elizabeth Scott, LCSW, and writer/former eating disorder sufferer Connie Sobczak founded The Body Positive to offer "a lively, healing community that offers freedom from suffocating societal messages that keep people in a perpetual struggle with their bodies."[14]

Body positivity urges us to accept our bodies, no matter what our sizes, shapes, skin tone, race, gender, or physical abilities, while we challenge socially accepted standards of beauty. If you have a healthy body image, you "feel comfortable in your body and you feel good about the way you look," according to the Office on Women's Health.[15]

Treat your body not like it's an ornament, but [like] it's a vehicle to your dreams.[16]

—**Taryn Brumfitt**, Australian writer/film director, body positivity advocate, and director of *Embrace: The Documentary*

Although I wrote this book to help you shed unhealthy excess pounds, I strongly embrace body positivity. Let me explain.

No matter what your present weight, I urge you to love, accept, and appreciate your body. Body positivity at its best, I contend, means taking great care of your wonderful body, moving it often, and feeding it nutritious foods so you can become happy, healthy, and energetic.

Let me leave you with an encouraging trend. In recent years, many people's priorities have shifted. According to more than one million people who took a Mayo Clinic Diet Assessment, 83 percent of participants were more motivated to improve their health than to lose weight for physical appearances.[17]

By now, I hope you, too, are driven by a desire to feel better, not just look better.

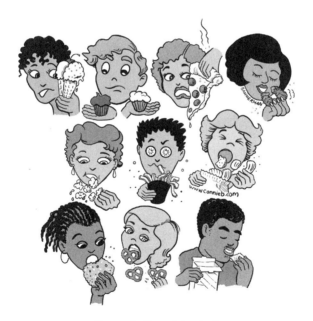

Do you do Stress Splurging?

Go to Your 21 Reasons List and Check Off Your Truth

It's time to take an objective look at your bingeing behavior when you're feeling anxious. Did you do Stress Splurging? If so, check Reason #9 on your 21 Reasons List.

Chapter 14

REASON #10

Why you blew your diet

You Crumpled under Peer Pressure from *Polite Food Pushers*

[T]he people who pressure you [to eat] do it out of love —they want you to share their food and the feelings that come with it. So it's hard to say no to peer pressure.[1]

—**Susan Albers, PsyD**, clinical psychologist at the Cleveland Clinic and author of *Hanger Management and Eating Mindfully*

Meals are times for togetherness and connection with friends and family. Studies even show that enjoying meals with your family or special people can provide benefits such as higher self-esteem, lower risk of depression, and greater satisfaction with your life.[2]

Sharing is all well and good, but your weight may swing up or down depending on the negative or positive influence of your spouse, friends, family members, or close coworkers.

Let's look at two ways peer pressure from these people—whom I refer to as *Polite Food Pushers* or *Subtle Enablers*—may derail your best intentions. You've decided to eat better and start the Bounce Back Diet. You excitedly tell your loved ones and friends. But they're not nearly as encouraging as you'd like.

To be fair, let's look at the situation from the perspective of those close to you. Over the years, your honey or buddies have seen you ditch one diet after another. They've watched your weight yo-yo up and down several times. Understandably, they're skeptical. They wrongly assume that this time, as before, you'll eventually return to eating sugary, fatty, carbs-rich junk foods. Of course, these folks mean well, but they may unknowingly belittle, delay, or disrupt your weight loss efforts.

When Your Loved Ones Are *Subtle Enablers*

Polite Food Pushers may not realize that they can doom or damage your chances of success. That's why you need to be prepared should you be met with skepticism, resistance, or dismissiveness.

The reality is that while you shed the pounds, you may receive very little support—if any—from your loved ones. Stanford University School of Medicine researchers found that more than 75 percent of people surveyed said they "never" or "rarely" got support from family or friends to shed weight.

According to the study in *Obesity*, 45.7 percent of female participants who "never" experienced family support were *least likely* to shed pounds. But women who got frequent friend and family support (approximately 71.6 percent) were *more likely* to release weight.[3]

Despite the lack of encouragement, 80 percent of the female participants still became "the most likely to lose weight." Why was that? The researchers speculated that "group-based programs provided support lacking from friendships."[4]

Polite Food Pushers or Subtle Enablers

These are well-meaning, possibly overweight or obese loved ones, friends, business colleagues, neighbors, or relatives who genially invite or pressure you to eat various sugary, salty, fatty, fried junk foods. These folks mean no harm when they insist that you try their fat-filled dishes. Like you, they've been raised to believe that food equals love, friendship, and good times. They want you to join in the fun. But their polite prodding can lead you to do *Peer Pressure Eating.* The good news? You can succeed without their support.

Your Honey May Thwart Your Weight Loss

You need to know that the biggest saboteur is usually the person closest to you. Research from Rutgers University found that your sweetheart can sabotage your weight loss when he or she brings home junk foods, urges you to cheat on your meal plan, tries to stop you from working out, makes hurtful comments, or even threatens to leave you.

"Romantic partners can stymie a significant other's weight loss goals by belittling their efforts and scrutinizing their efforts in ways that lead to hurt and conflict," the scientists wrote in their study, which was published in *Qualitative Health Research.*[5]

When dieters met resistance from their romantic partners, they stopped sharing their plans to shed weight. In addition, they became more likely to fail, the investigators discovered.

Other scholars writing in the *Journal of Health Psychology* aptly summed up the derisive attitude that weight-watching people may get from loved ones. The first part of the title tells it all: "Are you still on that stupid diet?"[6]

Unfortunately, when one partner loses weight, it may cause conflict, tension, nagging, resentment, and arguments about food or exercise. Significant others who didn't watch their weight felt threatened and insecure because of their partners' discipline and dieting success, according to a study in *Health Communication*. They acted out, made critical comments, lost interest in sex, or even encouraged the dieting partner to consume unhealthy foods.[7]

When "significant others resisted healthy changes and were not supportive of their partner's weight loss, the relationship suffered," explained Lynsey K. Romo, PhD, an associate professor of communication at North Carolina State University and lead author of the study.[8]

The research uncovered good news, too. "When both partners bought into the idea of healthy changes and were supportive of one another, weight loss appeared to bring people closer."

> *Nothing—not a conversation, not a handshake or even a hug—*
> *establishes friendship so forcefully as eating together.*[9]

> **—Jonathan Safran Foer**, novelist and bestselling
> author of *Everything Is Illuminated*

Choose Your Friends Carefully

Friends also can affect your weight. Consider:

- **Friends, especially female buddies, influence others' weight and health habits.** A review of sixteen studies, which looked at more than 22,000 males and females aged fourteen to seventy-three, found that friends affect each other's weight. The correlation was stronger in women, the researchers concluded in *Social Science and Medicine*. They also discovered that friends could just as easily influence each other to adopt *unhealthy habits* (such as eating fast food and skipping exercise) as *healthy habits* (eating better and getting fitter).[10]

- **Heavy people hang out with heavy friends.** Let's look at the conclusions from a landmark study published in the *New England Journal of Medicine*. After assessing more than 12,000 people for thirty-two years, researchers found that a person's chance of becoming obese increased by 57 percent if a close friend was obese, 40 percent if a sibling was obese, and 37 percent if the spouse was obese.[11]

- **Your partner or friends greatly influence your eating habits.**
  Additional insights came from University of California at Berkeley
  scientists, who followed more than 3,400 people for ten years. The
  study, which was published in the *American Journal of Public Health,*
  found that when it comes to overconsuming calories from snacks
  and alcohol, loved ones or friends can serve as either negative or
  positive influences.[12]

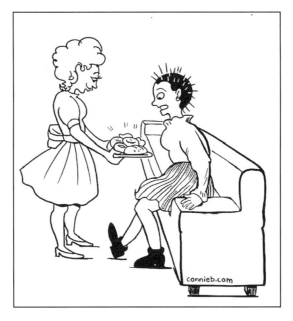

"P-l-e-a-s-e have some of my homemade cookies! If you don't, I'll be soooo hurt."

Have Your Closest Peeps Influenced You?

Now think about your loved ones and friends. Do they typically behave
like Polite Food Pushers or Subtle Enablers? Did they unknowingly lead
you to choose or overeat unhealthy foods? If you did Peer Pressure Eating,
check off #10 on your 21 Reasons List.

Chapter 15

REASON #11

Why you blew your diet

For Women Only: You Did *Time-of-Month* or *Time-of-Life Noshing*

*[At age 40,] you cannot eat the way you did
when you were 20. . . . If you continue to consume
the same amount of calories, by the age of 45, you can expect
to be 30 to 50 pounds heavier and at risk for health problems.*

*If you've been winging your diet up to this point,
the winging is over. You have to pay attention to what,
how much, and how often you eat. Period.*[1]

—**Pamela Peeke, MD, MPH**, assistant professor of medicine
at the University of Maryland School of Medicine and
author of *Fight Fat After Forty*

My dear ladies of all ages, we now come to a subject that's unique to us. When we seek to drop extra pounds or maintain weight, we need to be vigilant. Why? Our hormones.

Let's consider three different times in our lives when chocolate, fast carbs, or sweets may beckon. Choose which scenario holds true for you:

- **You're menstruating.** Do you crave sweet chocolate or other desserts in the week or so before your time of the month?
- **You gave birth up to six months ago.** Do you experience postpartum cravings?
- **You're going through or went through menopause, aka "the change."** Do you often desire sweets or processed carbs?

First let me share the good news: No matter what your age or stage of life, you'll find it easier to shed pounds or maintain your target weight when you eat a healthy diet that greatly reduces or eliminates processed sweets and quickie carbs.

Time-of-Month or Time-of-Life Noshing

That time of month (before menstruation) or time of life (after childbirth and/or during menopause and beyond) can be challenging. That's when urges for sweets, particularly chocolate, fast carbs, and junk foods, can come on strong. While caving into cravings is understandable, you need to know that indulging may cause your symptoms to get worse. But the fewer sweets or carbs you eat, the better you'll feel and the more stable your weight will become.

The Connection between Carbs or Sweets and PMS or Menopause Symptoms

Let's examine how eating sweets and high-glycemic carbs can affect two important stages of your life:

- **Consuming processed foods is connected to PMS symptoms.** A study published in *Nutrients* found that women who consumed a lot of calorie-loaded, sugary, fatty, salty foods were three times more likely to have symptoms of PMS, including muscle, joint, abdominal, and back pain. In addition, before their period, 84.7 percent of the females got food cravings, and 88.9 percent ate more sweets, especially chocolate and cake.[2]

- **High glycemic load increases the likelihood of PMS.** Research in *HealthMED* showed that "high carbohydrate intake may worsen premenstrual symptoms." The study cited a link between high glycemic load (the level of sugars flooding the bloodstream) and PMS in students who were big consumers of refined carbs.[3]

- **The worse your PMS, the more you'll overeat.** A study in the *Journal of Pediatric and Adolescent Gynecology* looked at women with disordered eating symptoms and PMS symptoms ranging from mild to debilitating. The researchers noticed that "as the severity of premenstrual symptoms increase, disordered eating behaviors also increase."[4]

Meanwhile, when you're in menopause or perimenopause, you also may be more vulnerable to cravings and piling on pounds because your metabolism slows down when your estrogen and progesterone levels decrease. Learn more from these studies:

- **The more processed carbs you eat, the worse your symptoms.** During menopause, the more refined carbs you eat, the more you may experience such symptoms as weight gain, a slower metabolism, hot flashes, chills, night sweats, mood changes, vaginal dryness, and sleep problems, according to a study in *Maturitas: An international journal of midlife and beyond*. The opposite held true as well. "Higher fiber intake, lower intake of liquid carbohydrates and a lower value of the dietary glycemic index are associated with lower rates of hot flashes and night sweats during menopause," the researchers learned.[5]

- **Women in their 40s and 50s with higher blood sugar levels have more frequent hot flashes.** For eight years, researchers studied more than 3,000 women aged forty-two to fifty-two. Those with higher blood sugar levels (from eating more sweets and processed carbs) had more frequent hot flashes irrespective of their weight or estrogen levels, according to a study in *The Journal of Clinical Endocrinology and Metabolism.*[6]

> *It became so apparent to me that after I ate rich chocolaty things, I would get very warm, start perspiring, and become crabby and more impatient.*
>
> *Sugar was triggering hot flashes, interrupting my sleep, making me spacey and forgetful, and causing volatility in my personality . . . It became easy for me to say that the chocolate just was not worth it.*[7]
>
> **—Kathy Smith,** fitness expert and bestselling author of *Kathy Smith's Moving Through Menopause* and other books

When You're Pregnant or after You Give Birth (Time of Life)

Ladies, being pregnant isn't a reason to overeat because you're now eating for two. However, close to 50 percent of pregnant women gained more weight than recommended by official guidelines, according to the *American Journal of Obstetrics and Gynecology.*[8]

After you've delivered a baby, the pregnancy pounds will come off more easily if you avoid simple sugars and carbs and eat nutrient-dense foods. You also may lose weight more quickly if you're breastfeeding because you'll burn about 500 extra calories a day.[9]

Postpartum weight retention is an important predictor of long-term obesity and type 2 diabetes. Indeed, research shows that new mothers who fail to lose the pregnancy pounds are at increased risk for obesity later in life, according to research in the *American Journal of Preventive Medicine.*[10]

No Matter What Your Time of Life, When You Eat Healthier Foods, You'll Be Healthier

Now be heartened by these promising results:

- **Replacing sweets and processed carbs with more wholesome foods led to fewer PMS Symptoms.** Research published in *Public Health Nutrition* found that women whose diets were high in fast foods, soft drinks, sweets, and desserts struggled more with

PMS symptoms. On the other hand, those who ate more whole foods (including vegetables, legumes, fruits, nuts, garlic, fish, pickles, and yogurt) were more likely to breeze though the month with little or no PMS symptoms.[11]

- **New mothers who ate fewer carbs lost more weight postpartum.** A study in the journal *Food & Function* found that new moms who ate a mostly low-carb, low–glycemic load diet with high protein and fat intake from animal sources had significantly lower body weight at one-year postpartum, compared to women who consumed more carbs.[12]

- **For menopausal women, curtailing carbs reduced symptoms and decreased weight gain.** After examining data from more than 88,000 postmenopausal women aged forty-nine to eighty-one, investigators found that a reduced-carbohydrate diet with moderate fat and high protein intake was the most effective way to reduce weight gain after menopause, according to a study in the *British Journal of Nutrition*. Women who took in about one-third of their daily calories from carbs had the lowest risk of gaining weight after one year, compared to those following either a Mediterranean-style diet, a low-fat plan, or one consistent with USDA guidelines. (By the way, this research suggested that a low-fat diet may *promote* rather than *prevent* weight gain after menopause.[13])

The facts are clear. No matter what your time of month or time of life, eating fewer and better carbs, as well as ample protein and sufficient quality fat, will lessen your cravings, lower your insulin levels, balance your blood sugar levels, and reduce belly fat.

Now think about your eating habits around that time of month or life. Did you turn to more carbs or sweets during one of those scenarios? If so, mark a check next to #11 on your 21 Reasons List.

Chapter 16

REASON #12

Why you blew your diet

You Succumbed to *Mindless Munching*

When we don't fully concentrate on our meals and the process of taking in food, we fall into a trap of mindless eating where we don't track or recognize the food that has just been consumed.[1]

—Jane Ogden, PhD, health psychologist and lead author of a study about on-the-go eaters

You stroll through the supermarket for your weekly shopping trip. As you make your way through the grocery store, you quickly toss more and more things into your shopping cart.

Finally, while you wait impatiently at the check-out stand, the cashier keeps ringing up one thing after another, and your eyes get bigger and bigger as your bill goes higher and higher.

Oh goodness! Somehow, to your shock, your shopping cart is piled high with sugar-carbs-and-salt-filled junk foods.

Later that day or evening, many of these foods find their way into your belly. Frankly, you don't know how it happened.

Now, it's one thing to mindlessly graze and gorge when you're kicking back at home, going out socially, or buying food, but if you're also overcome by grief, trauma, or stress, or you're going through that time of month or life, watch out!

That's when your eating may escalate into what I consider Mindless Munching.

With this type of bingeing, you generally don't notice how much or what you're eating. You zone out. Then, somehow—you're not sure how—you may devour monstrous amounts of crackers, cookies, or carbage in only five to fifteen minutes.

When you go automatic, Mindless Munching can whoosh in quickly. Your bingeing takes on a life of its own. You can absent-mindedly put away hundreds, possibly thousands of calories.

The problem with fast, inattentive eating is that your belly doesn't have time to catch up with your fast-working hands and rapid-fire teeth. Remember, your stomach needs up to twenty minutes before it receives "I'm full" signals from your brain.[2]

Those twenty minutes are pivotal because, during that all-important time, you can easily ditch the diet.

Mindless Munching

Mindless Munching is when you inattentively, unthinkingly stuff your face with carbage, sweets, fast foods, or other nutrient-lacking junk foods. When you become distracted, careless, or oblivious to what you're doing, you can unknowingly inhale a large bag of chips, a gallon of ice cream, or a family-sized package of cookies within minutes. This type of overeating can go hand-in-hand with binge-watching, Heartbreak Bingeing, Divorce Devouring, or Blood Sugar Rollercoaster Scarfing.

How Mindless Munching Triggers Weight Gain

Compelling research reveals how not paying attention to what, where, how much, or how fast you're eating can be damaging to your waistline. Consider:

- **Looking at your smartphone while eating may lead to weight gain.** A study published in *Physiology & Behavior* found that people who used their smartphones while eating consumed 15 percent more calories than when they weren't staring at their devices.[3]
- **Eating while watching TV, reading, or being distracted may result in eating more now *and* later.** A review of twenty-four studies published in the *American Journal of Clinical Nutrition* found that not paying attention during a meal (being distracted by TV, radio, or reading) led subjects to eat more food at that meal *and* later in the day, compared with people who focused on their food while eating.[4]
- **Eating quickly can make you bigger.** Scientists who pooled results from twenty-three studies found a correlation between how fast people ate and how big they were. The study in the *International Journal of Obesity* discovered that folks who ate quickly were 2.2 times more likely to be obese than those who ate slowly.[5]

Did I describe your pattern(s)? Do you do Mindless Munching? If so, make a check in front of Reason #12 on your 21 Reasons List.

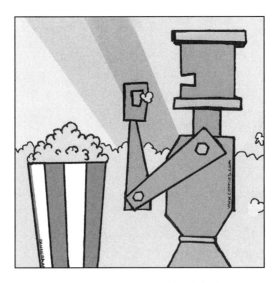

Are you a Mindless-Munching Robot?

Chapter 17

REASONS #13 to 21

why you blew your diet

You Skimped on Sleep, Sat Too Much, Skipped Sunshine, or Made Other Unhealthy Lifestyle Choices

*For years, I drank eight to 12 cans of diet soda every day.
I was overweight, had developed terrible adult acne and my energy
[was low]. When I [tried] to get healthy, I saw doctors,
tried diets, and started counting calories, but nothing worked.*

*When I finally decided to swap my diet soda for plain water
as a test, I couldn't believe the results. I lost over 20 pounds,
my skin cleared up, and my energy was back.[1]*

—**Kara Goldin,** founder and former CEO of Hint and
bestselling author of *Undaunted: Overcoming Doubts & Doubters*

Let's wrap up our examination of why you've been eating badly. While you read this chapter, remember to keep your 21 Reasons List handy so you can keep track of your unhealthy habits.

REASON #13

You Skimped on Sleep

Adults over age eighteen need seven or more hours of sleep each night, but one in three Americans don't get enough zzzs.[2]

You may be sleep-deprived if you spend lots of time online, play video games, binge-watch your favorite shows right before bedtime, or keep your cell phone next to your bed while you slumber. All these activities can keep you wired and awake, because electronic gadgets emit an excess of blue light that throws off your circadian rhythm. (That's the internal process that regulates your sleep-wake cycle over about twenty-four hours.[3])

An overwhelming body of research has established
the links between lack of sleep and weight gain.[4]

—Michael J. Breus, PhD, clinical psychologist and author of
the *Sleep Doctor's Diet Plan: Lose Weight through Better Sleep*

The connection between insufficient sleep and weight gain has been confirmed by study after study:

- **Sleep deprivation may lead to junk food cravings.** When researchers looked at brain scans of young adults after a sleepless night and then again after a full night's rest, they found that parts of the brain linked with reward and cravings fired up after the sleepless nights. The study in *Nature Communications* concluded that sleep deprivation may be linked to cravings for junk foods such as donuts, pizza, and burgers, all of which can cause weight gain.[5]

- **Less than seven hours of sleep causes higher levels of obesity.** People who slept less than seven hours per night were 40 percent more likely to develop obesity than people who got zzzs for longer, according to findings published in *BMJ Open Sport and Exercise Medicine*. Researchers found that lack of sleep also was linked with the hunger hormone ghrelin. In addition, sleep deprivation was associated with lower insulin sensitivity and decreased levels of leptin, the hormone that helps regulate food intake.[6]

- **Stress leads to poor sleep, which can cause uncontrolled eating.** Those who slept poorly demonstrated a greater tendency toward uncontrolled eating and overeating based on comfort rather than physical hunger, according to a study in *Nutrients*. When the subjects got their stress under control, they slept better and didn't overeat as much.[7]

Did sleep deprivation cause you to eat poorly? If so, check off #13 on your 21 Reasons List.

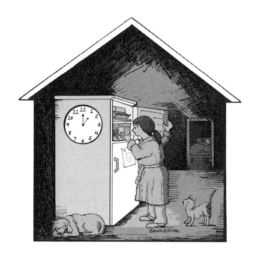

"I hope my family doesn't catch me raiding the fridge again!"

REASON #14

You Ate Late at Night

Do you snack or eat late dinners within an hour or two of bedtime? If so, that may be another reason you packed on pounds. Research shows that eating close to bedtime is problematic:

- **If you eat late, you eat more.** A study in *Nutrition Research* looked at meal timing and calorie intake in subjects. The researchers observed that people who ate dinner closer to their bedtime consumed more calories overall than those who consumed their last meal four hours earlier.[8]

- **If you eat more at night, you may have trouble sleeping.** A study published in *Journal of Clinical Sleep Medicine* found that eating more heavily at night was associated with a deterioration in several measurements of sleep quality.[9]
- **When you eat a late dinner, you burn less fat and have higher blood sugar levels.** Research published in the *Journal of Clinical Endocrinology* showed that people who ate dinner an hour before bedtime burned less fat and had higher blood sugar levels than when they had the same meal five hours before bedtime.[10]

If you're a late-night eater, check #14 on your 21 Reasons List.

REASON #15
You Sat Too Much

Millions of us spend too much time lying on the couch, sitting on our butts, and being sedentary. You may think that getting the recommended thirty minutes of exercise a day or 150 minutes a week is enough to counteract the negative effects of remaining on your rear end for hours, but that's not true. Even if you exercise most days, you still want to move your body often throughout the day and evening.

Another problem with staying on your fanny for hours on end is that it may be conducive to poor food choices. After sitting for a long time, you may feel lethargic, sluggish, or unmotivated to eat properly—especially when your kitchen or work vending machines are within easy reach. Now for more research:

- **Sedentary people preferred high-calorie, high-fat junk foods.** A study published in *Medicine & Science in Sports & Exercise* revealed that sedentary people had a higher desire for high-calorie, high-fat junk foods than those who started working out regularly on a treadmill.[11]

The opposite holds true, too.

- **People who take breaks from sitting eat better.** Investigators writing in *BMJ Open* discovered that public school teachers who took the most breaks from sitting during the day ate more nutritious foods such as fruits and vegetables.[12]

Do you sit too much? If so, jot down yes next to Reason #15 on your list.

REASON #16

You "Rewarded" Yourself with Junk Foods after Exercising

You put in a rigorous exercise session. Great! But then did you feel that you deserved a "reward" such as a large portion of spaghetti, a piece of cake, or a glass of wine? Not so fast! Physical activity doesn't undo overeating.

- **"Treating yourself" after working out can backfire.** A study in the *Journal of Physical Activity and Health* found that food played an important role as a reward after exercise. After working out, the subjects felt that they could treat themselves with something special, such as eating at a fast-food restaurant.[13]

What about you? Do you "treat" yourself with cunning carbs or a high-calorie snack after working out? If this is your pattern, make a check mark next to Reason #16 on your list.

REASON #17

You Consumed Artificial Sweeteners

Are you one of 41 percent of American adults who consume diet foods or beverages containing artificial sweeteners?[14] If so, that may be another reason you blew your diet.

In fact, I invite you to question the claim from the American Beverage Association (ABA), the trade association that represents manufacturers of nonalcoholic beverages in the United States. The ABA contends that the "current body of available science shows that low- and no-calorie sweeteners can help reduce calories consumed and aid in maintaining a healthy weight."[15]

Instead, I suggest that you consider another theory. Although artificial sweeteners, such as saccharin (Sweet'N Low), acesulfame potassium (Sweet One), aspartame (Equal or NutraSweet), neotame (Newtame), and sucralose (Splenda) are low in calories, some scientists liken them to a Trojan horse that tricks your taste buds and fools your brain. For instance:

- **Research found a link between artificial sweeteners and weight gain.** A review of more than 406,000 people published in the *Canadian Medical Association Journal* analyzed data from thirty-seven investigations and found an association between consuming artificial sweeteners and "relatively higher risks" of weight gain and obesity, high blood pressure, type 2 diabetes, heart disease, metabolic syndrome, and other health issues.[16]

- **People shed more weight when they switched from diet drinks to water.** A study in the *American Journal of Clinical Nutrition* found that participants did better at shedding pounds when they drank H_2O instead of diet drinks. The water drinkers lost an average of 2.6 pounds more in 24 weeks than those who downed diet drinks, losing 19.4 pounds versus 16.8 pounds.[17]

Interestingly, the World Health Organization (WHO) released guidelines in May 2023 that recommend against consuming nonsugar sweeteners to control body weight. The advice was based on the findings of a review that suggests these non-nutritive sweeteners don't provide any long-term benefits in reducing body fat in adults or children. In the study, the researchers also speculated that long-term use of artificial sweeteners may lead to an increased risk of type 2 diabetes, cardiovascular diseases, and mortality in adults.[18]

What's your pattern? Do you drink beverages with artificial sweeteners or eat foods containing them? If yes, indicate so next to Reason #17 on your list.

REASON #18

You Drank Too Little Water

This may seem counterintuitive, but your body releases excess water when you're adequately hydrated. But if you don't drink enough water, your body holds onto what little water it has, not knowing when more is coming. Insufficient H_2O can lead to weight gain, bloating, and fluid retention.[19] Check out these findings:

- **Women who drank more water shed body fat and weren't as hungry.** Overweight women made *only one change* to their daily regimen. They drank six additional glasses of water each day, splitting it into two cups before breakfast, before lunch, and before dinner. After eight weeks, the water-drinkers shed on average 3.2 pounds and had reduced hunger levels, according to a study published in the *Journal of Natural Science, Biology and Medicine*.[20]
- **People who drink ample water maintain a healthy weight.** A study published in the *Annals of Family Medicine* found that peo-

ple who didn't get enough water had higher odds of being obese as compared to hydrated adults.[21]

What's your daily water intake? Go to your list and check off Reason #18 if you think not drinking enough H^2O may have contributed to your weight gain.

REASON #19

You Had a Nightcap or More

Another major diet wrecker is alcohol, which can add empty calories and lower your inhibitions. If you have a couple of glasses of wine, beer, or a cocktail, you're more likely to cast aside your good intentions to eat healthy foods. Consider:

- **Reducing alcohol may help with weight loss.** A study in *Appetite* found that cutting back on booze seems "warranted, particularly for individuals with high levels of impulsivity."[22]
- **Evidence suggests that booze may disrupt sleep.** Alcohol may affect sleep quality, especially the period of rapid eye movement, or REM, sleep. (REM sleep—when dreaming occurs—plays an important role in memory, learning, emotional processing, and brain development.)[23] And recall that inadequate sleep can lead to weight gain.

Now go to Reason #19 and notate if regularly drinking alcohol is one of your habits, which may have led to weight gain.

REASON #20

You Didn't Get Enough Vitamin D, the Sunshine Vitamin

The link between vitamin D deficiency and weight gain and obesity is well documented. In fact, nearly 42 percent of people are estimated to have a vitamin D deficiency, according to a study in *Nutrition Research*.[24] Let's look at some Sunshine Vitamin research:

- **Vitamin D deficiency was found in obese and overweight people.** A review in the journal *Obesity Reviews* discovered that vitamin D deficiency was 35 percent higher in obese subjects and 24 percent higher in the overweight group.[25]

- **Supplementing with vitamin D promoted weight loss.** For a study published in the *American Journal of Clinical Nutrition,* researchers put overweight and obese women on a calorie-restricted diet and exercise routine. Half the participants took a vitamin D supplement of 2,000 IU, and the other half swallowed a placebo. After one year, the women supplementing with vitamin D lost an average of 7 pounds more than those who didn't take the supplement.[26]

To get enough Vitamin D, you want to expose your face, arms, and legs to the sun for fifteen to thirty minutes without sunscreen at least twice a week between 10 a.m. and 4 p.m., as the National Institutes of Health's Office of Dietary Supplements recommends.[27] The rest of the time you're outside, wear sunscreen.

If you live in a part of the country where the sun doesn't shine much certain times of year, the Endocrine Society recommends supplementing with 400 to 1,000 IU of vitamin D per day.[28] You also can get your vitamin D levels checked by your doctor to get more personalized advice.

By the way, vitamin D doesn't come from sunshine alone. It also naturally occurs in such foods as trout, salmon, sardines, tuna, mackerel, fish liver oils, and egg yolks.[29]

Do you regularly get enough vitamin D from sunshine, food, or supplements? If not, make a check next to Reason #20 on your list.

REASON #21

You're Stuck in the *Not-Enough Syndrome*

For the final reason you blew your diet, you want to take a good look at yourself, your priorities, and how you spend your time. Are you leading a well-balanced life? Or are you trapped by what I call the *Not-Enough Syndrome*? If you're not getting what you need and want, you probably felt discouraged, frustrated, or unfulfilled. Those exasperating feelings may have led you to overeat.

For instance, do you have ample love, joy, laughter, friends, hobbies, or fun? Would you like to work less and play more? Would you love to spend more time doing things you love?

Do you yearn for more "me time" to read good books, play pickleball, or take up gardening? Would you like to spend more quality time with your kid(s)? Would you love weekly date nights with your sweetie? What about that long-overdue vacation? Have you put off a big dream?

Think now about those things you really want. Does what I'm saying ring true for you? Have you been trapped by the Not-Enough Syndrome? If so, check off Reason #21 on your list.

You May Have Other Reasons You Ate Badly

You've now learned what I've identified as 21 Reasons You Blew Your Diet. Bear in mind, though, that I haven't listed every reason people eat badly. For instance, I didn't delve into any health conditions or medications that may affect your appetite and your weight.

I'm eager to hear your thoughts. Which of the 21 Reasons ring a bell? If you think I left out other reasons people blew their diets, please let me know. Just e-mail me through my website at www.BounceBackDiet.com.

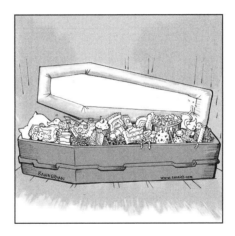

Junk foods belong in the coffin!

You Now Know Why You Blew Your Diet

Way to go! High fives to you for bravely exploring 21 Reasons You Blew Your Diet and then deciding which ones apply to you.

It's time to review. Look at all the items you checked off on this list. How many reasons were relevant to you? What did you discover? Did any patterns emerge? What unhealthy habits can you change? Journal about your realizations.

Now let me officially congratulate you. Finally—after years of confusion, discouragement, and exasperation—you have a good grasp of why you blew your diet.

You're ready to move on to the next phase of our transformational journey together. You're ready to Bounce Back Boldly.

Part III

Take Back Your Power

The
Bounce Back
Boldly
Plan

*Once you make a decision,
the Universe conspires to make it happen.*[1]
—Ralph Waldo Emerson (1803–1882),
visionary and poet

105

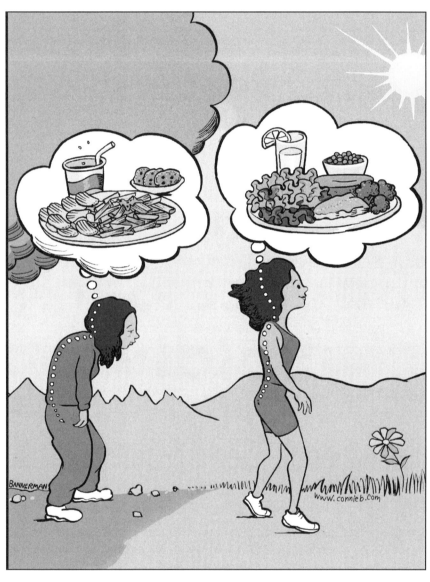

You can Flip On Your Success Mindset.

Chapter 18

Flip On Your
Success Mindset

At various points, in big ways and small,
we get knocked down. If we stay down,
grit loses. If we get up, grit prevails.[1]

—Angela Duckworth, PhD, psychologist and
New York Times bestselling author of
Grit: The Power of Passion and Perseverance

Now that you understand why you blew your diet, you're ready to pump up your motivation, heal your heart, and create happy, healthy, harmonious habits. All the while, you'll release excess pounds while you lovingly respect your precious, one-and-only body by feeding it nutritious foods.

To truly grasp how massively you'll transform, let's look at the definition of the phrase *bounce back*. According to *Merriam-Webster Dictionary*, this means you'll "return quickly to a normal condition after a difficult situation or event."[2]

The *Collins Dictionary* further explains that when you "bounce back after a bad experience," you achieve "your previous level of success, enthusiasm, or activity."[3]

But you want to set your sights much higher. Vanilla-flavored bouncing back isn't nearly enough. Your mission is to outpace the old you.

Your goal is to Bounce Back with passion, pizazz, and purpose. You'll harness your bravery, confidence, and determination. Indeed, you'll reinvent yourself while you become healthier, stronger, and more resilient.

To capture this feeling of becoming better and better, I added the word *boldly*, which means that you're "showing or requiring a fearless, daring spirit."[4] Likewise, it signifies that you're assured, confident, adventurous, and free.

In short, you're on your way. You'll now learn proven tactics to *Bounce Back Boldly.*

Bounce Back Boldly

You've been through some trying times, and, as a result, you mindlessly binged on sweets, carbage, and/or fast foods for weeks, months, or years, and packed on a few or a lot of unwanted pounds. While eating badly, you also lost your power, got stuck in a rut, and became less than you can be.

Now, to reinvent yourself, take command of your life, and drop excess weight, you're taking a two-pronged approach. First, you're following the Bounce Back Boldly Plan using evidence-based Fast, Easy, Awesome, Simple, Tested Strategies (FEASTS) that help you heal your heart, claim calm quickly, and shift from powerless to powerful. At the same time, you'll eat clean, wholesome, energy-dense, blood-sugar-balanced, modified ketogenic (KetoMod) foods while you follow the Bounce Back Diet. When you tackle the plan and diet at the same time, you'll be on track to becoming the remarkable person you can be.

Weight Loss (or Any Change) Begins in Your Mind

Before you begin to put better foods in your belly, you want to fill yourself up with empowering beliefs, dreams, and thoughts.

Indeed, your healthier, fitter body and loftier state of mind start to materialize when you imagine how you'd like to feel, look, and act. That's why you're first supercharging your attitude with positivity and possibility.

To help you go all in on this theory, know that you can Flip On Your Success Mindset just as easily as you turn on a light switch.

> *Change of diet will not help a man who will not change his thoughts. When a man makes his thoughts pure, he no longer desires impure food.*[5]

> **—James Allen** (1864–1912), author of the inspirational classic, *As a Man Thinketh*

Let's now dive into five simple steps to activate a rosy perspective:

DESIRE

We can discover the first step to achieve anything we want from Napoleon Hill's landmark bestseller *Think and Grow Rich*, whose enduring wisdom holds true decades after its 1937 publication.[6]

"A burning desire to be, and to do, is the starting point from which the dreamer must take off," explained Hill, who devoted more than twenty years interviewing 500 plus self-made industry titans of his time to unearth tried-and-true principles of success.[7]

What does your *burning desire* for a healthier, stronger body feel like for you?

Go deep into what it feels like. Excitedly step into your fabulous body. Are you:

- Overjoyed that you can easily touch your toes, walk three miles, and feel healthier, fitter, and more flexible than when you were a teen?
- Grinning proudly when your surprised doctor announces that you have reached your target weight *and* that one or more pressing medical conditions have vanished?

- Bursting with more energy than you've had for years—so much so that you want to romp in bed with your sweetie, who's delighted by your sudden stamina? (You know what I mean. Hey, this is a PG-13 book.)

Continue to nurture your burning desire so that it becomes an "all-consuming obsession," Hill suggested.[8]

> *Your life changes the moment you make a new,*
> *congruent, and committed decision.*[9]

—**Tony Robbins**, master motivator and *New York Times* bestselling author of *Unshakeable* and others

DECIDE

Next, to manifest your healthier, stronger, sexier body, you want to *decide* that you will succeed. No ifs, ands, or buts about it.

When you emphatically decide to shed excess pounds, your self-limiting beliefs melt away. Your firm resolve sparks a friendly invisible force that speeds you to success. Your decisive commitment liberates you and leads you to behave in ways aligned with your goals.

For instance, if you see fattening foods at a store or party, your burning desire and definite decision to let go of excess fat to become healthy will guide you to effortlessly ignore those junky edibles and instead joyously choose healthier foods for your amazing body.

> *When you constantly expect that which you persistently desire, your*
> *ability to attract becomes irresistible. Desire connects you with the thing*
> *desired and expectation draws it into your life. This is the Law.*[10]

—**Raymond Holliwell** (1900–1986), author of
Working with the Law: 11 Truth Principles for Successful Living

EXPECT

Now you want to know without a shadow of a doubt that you'll be triumphant, *no matter what,* at shedding unhealthy excess pounds—or, for that matter, accomplishing whatever goal you set. You want to expect success in every fiber of your being.

"Expectancy is like a magnet, drawing to you experiences that you would love," explains dream-building expert Mary Morrissey, who has devoted more than four decades to teaching and studying transformation.[11]

Then go even further. "Turn up the volume of your expectancy, and feel that [your success] is real with absolute certainty," urges Morrissey, author of the inspiring book *Brave Thinking: The Art and Science of Creating a Life You Love*.[12]

"Whatever image your mind clings to will tend to replicate itself in your real world," she insists.

VISUALIZE

We now come to the powerful process of visualization. This is when you repeatedly see what you desire (weight loss and good health in this instance) *as if it has already happened*. You can think of visualization as purposeful daydreaming, intentional fantasizing, or positive imagining. The point is that you want to have a clear picture of the future you who *already achieved* your cherished dreams.

If envisioning what you want feels a little woo-woo, you need to know that peer-reviewed scientific research has validated the effectiveness of visualization:[13]

- Students have applied visualization to improve their grades.[14]
- Surgeons have used it before they perform operations.[15]
- Stroke patients have practiced positive imagining to regain movement in affected limbs.[16]
- Visualization has helped tennis players relieve stress.[17]
- Mental imagery has minimized depression and anxiety.[18]
- Seeing a goal achieved in advance can be a powerful motivator to complete a race or finish a task.[19]

Harvard-trained psychiatrist and brain-imaging researcher Srini Pillay, MD, describes how imagining your desired outcome works.

"It is now a well-known fact that we stimulate the same brain regions when we visualize an action and when we actually perform that same action," Dr. Pillay explained to me.[20]

"Imagery warms up the brain's movement centers, allowing you to reach your goals more effortlessly. Not knowing 'how' doesn't actually matter as much as we might think it does since the brain will figure this out once you let it know where you want to go," he amplified.

> *I would visualize things coming to me that I wanted. . . . It just made me feel better. I would drive home and think, 'Well, I do have these things; they're out there, I just don't have ahold of them yet. . . . [Visualization is] about letting the universe know what you want and then [working] towards it while letting go of how it comes to pass.*[21]

—**Jim Carrey**, who, while a struggling actor, reportedly wrote himself a $10 million check for "acting services rendered," dated it several years in the future, and in 1995 received that exact amount to star in the film *Dumb and Dumber*

Visualization is so remarkably effective that a host of mega-successful people—including business titan Oprah Winfrey, singer Lady Gaga, and Spanx founder Sarah Blakely—credit the practice with helping them achieve their goals.[22]

Interestingly, the act of seeing yourself succeed gained momentum thanks to stellar golfer Tiger Woods, basketball player Michael Jordan, and swimmer Michael Phelps.[23]

"Visualizing just mentally prepares you," remarks Phelps, the most decorated Olympian, who won a whopping twenty-eight gold medals.[24]

"Once you put yourself in a relaxed state, it's like watching a movie," explains Bob Bowman, the long-time trainer for Phelps.[25]

"The key to visualization," he adds, is that "number one, it has to be very vivid" and "it has to be rehearsed many, many times . . . because the brain cannot distinguish between something that's really vividly visualized and something that's real."

Visualizing your goals coming true "activates the law of attraction, programs your brain to achieve your dreams, and builds your internal motivation to take the necessary actions to achieve your dreams," explains Jack Canfield, who with coauthor Mark Victor Hansen, imagined spectacular success for their book *Chicken Soup for the Soul,* even when 144 publishers passed on publishing it.[26]

Despite a slew of rejections, the persistent authors kept seeing their book become a major bestseller. Ultimately, that first *Chicken Soup for the*

Soul book spawned a series of more than 275 titles, which have sold in excess of 500 million copies worldwide.

So how do you visualize? "Put yourself in the picture," suggests Mike Dooley, metaphysical teacher and the *New York Times* bestselling author of *Infinite Possibilities: The Art of Living Your Dreams.*[27]

"Consider and include every conceivable detail. See the sights, hear the sounds, smell the aromas, feel the textures. When you visualize, always go straight to the end result or beyond.

"Never ever mess with the cursed *hows*," Dooley insists. "They're the domain of the universe."

Science Shows That Visualization Promotes Weight Loss

Can visualizing help you release extra weight? You bet! Let's consider research published in the *International Journal of Obesity*, which showed that personalized, goal-directed mental imagery or visualization can help you peel off pounds, especially when you anticipate potential obstacles and mentally try out solutions that previously worked.[28]

For the study, researchers recruited 141 overweight or obese people with a BMI over twenty-five. One group of subjects received "Functional Imagery Training" (FIT), which incorporates visualization. The others participated in "Motivational Interviewing" (MI), a tactic that uses verbal coaching but *no* visual strategies.

All subjects took part in an initial in-person session, a phone follow-up, booster calls every two weeks for three months, monthly calls for six months, and four hours of consulting.

Mind you, all subjects were *never told* what or how much to eat or to work out. They didn't even get weight-loss coaching. Instead, they discussed their goals, recorded them on logs, and shared their motivations for losing weight with therapists who instructed them how to use guided imagery, along with a goal-directed app.

Now pay close attention. A year later, *the visualizers* (who vividly imagined their success) scored a weight loss of *more than fourteen pounds!* But those who didn't do any envisioning shed less than 1.5 pounds.

That's not all. The imaginers also took off more than three and a half inches from their waist circumference as opposed to the non-visualizers, who released less than one inch.

Why did the visualizers succeed so spectacularly? To find out, I reached out to head researcher Jackie Andrade, PhD, a professor in the School of Psychology at the University of Plymouth in the United Kingdom.

Participants "fully immersed themselves" in the fantasy of the experience using "multisensory imagery," Dr. Andrade clarified.[29]

"It is really important that the person feels what it would be like to do X, emotionally, rather than just picturing it."

Participants in the FIT group also were encouraged to imagine *the pleasure they'd get* while taking steps toward their goal and after they achieved it. For instance, they were invited to feel *the satisfaction* they'd get by attending the gym or walking instead of driving to work.

The study subjects also were instructed to imagine detailed "episodic imagery" in which they "anticipated problematic situations, as well as planned and rehearsed effective responses to them," Dr. Andrade added.

To summarize, the successful subjects visually *imagined that they already had achieved* their weight loss goals, and they saw themselves overcoming any challenges.

Sure enough, they successfully peeled off pounds just as they'd visualized.

Affirmations are statements going beyond the reality of the present into the creation of the future through the words you use in the now.[30]

—Louise L. Hay (1926–2017), manifestation guru, *New York Times* bestselling author of *You Can Heal Your Life,* and founder of Hay House

AFFIRM

Your last step to Flip On Your Success Mindset is to emphatically and joyfully repeat positive affirmations that harness the power of *autosuggestion*.[31] That's when you give positive instructions to your subconscious mind. Doing so will reprogram you to build your faith, boost your morale, and believe in your ability to succeed.[32]

Make sure that when you visualize and repeat affirmations, you *really* feel the joy, excitement, and elation as if you already had achieved your goal.

"All thoughts which have been emotionalized (given feeling) and mixed with faith, begin immediately to translate themselves into their physical equivalent," Napoleon Hill explains.[33]

"Emotion is the turbo charger of manifestation," adds manifestation expert Dooley. "It makes the whole process happen faster."[34]

While you visualize success and repeat affirmations, you want to have faith that you'll achieve your goals. Naturally, if you like, you can pray to God or Universal Intelligence (however you see this divine entity). Indeed, you can build faith no matter what your religious beliefs, even if you're an atheist or agnostic.

> *[W]ith a little faith, people can fix things, and they truly can change, because at that moment, you could not believe otherwise.*[35]

—**Mitch Albom**, journalist, broadcaster, and author of the *New York Times* bestselling books *Have a Little Faith* and *Tuesdays with Morrie*

Choose and State Affirmations That Declare Your Awesomeness

Before you begin to think about melting away fat, you want to proclaim to yourself and to the universe how truly wonderful you are. Infuse your statements with positive emotions. Cheerfully, confidently, triumphantly repeat your empowering affirmations whenever you can.

Declare your affirmations out loud with oomph and excitement first thing in the morning. Joyfully repeat them. Assert that they're true while you prepare meals, take a shower, or get dressed for success.

If other people are around, just repeat your affirmative statements silently or under your breath, or say them quietly while you go for a walk, take a bike ride, or do grocery shopping. In short, your affirmations can accompany and inspire you as you go about your day.

Here are five affirmations to help put you in a positive frame of mind for any endeavor:

Starter Affirmations to Bounce Back Boldly

I am awesome, bold, and confident.

Every day, in every way, I am happier, healthier, and stronger.

I am the amazing person I know I can be.

I am treating my body with love and respect.

I am in love with myself and my precious body.

Quick Refresher: How to Flip On Your Success Mindset

Let's recap. Every day, repeat these simple but powerful steps.

- **DESIRE** deeply (i.e., nurture a burning desire backed by faith) to be healthy, energetic, and at the best weight for your height and frame.
- **DECIDE** that you'll be triumphant at shedding extra weight no matter what.
- **EXPECT** success with absolute certainty.
- **VISUALIZE** that you've already claimed your fine, fit, flexible body.
- **AFFIRM** your new truths often by confidently and joyfully repeating positive declarations that unleash the power of autosuggestion.

To remember this five-part sequence to Flip On Your Success Mindset, just think of the acronym DDEVA (for Desire Decide Expect Visualize Affirm).

As you may have noticed, DDEVA coincidentally rhymes with "diva," the Latin word for goddess. Bear in mind, of course, that we're using DDEVA in a flattering way.

Now keep these mindset-shifting principles at the forefront of your consciousness while you jump-start your adventure to Bounce Back Boldly.

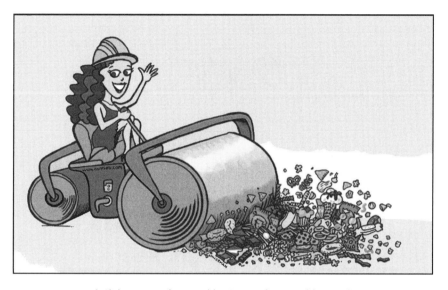

Let's have some fun smashing temptation to smithereens!

Beyond-the-Book Support:
Get My DDEVA Gift

For an easy recap of the five DDEVA steps to Flip On Your Success Mindset, I've created a helpful PDF. Print out a copy to put on your desk, attach to your fridge or bathroom mirror, and place near your bed so you'll get frequent reminders of your pleasing vision. Get your download at <u>www.BounceBackDiet.com/Book-Bonuses</u>.

Chapter 19

Week One

THE BOUNCE BACK
BOLDLY PLAN

*If one advances confidently in the direction of his dreams,
and endeavors to live the life which he has imagined, he will
meet with a success unexpected in common hours.*[1]

—Henry David Thoreau (1817–1862), naturalist,
poet, philosopher, and author of *Walden*

DAY 1

NUDGE YOURSELF TO EAT BETTER

Dump the doughnuts and chaos
and watch the clock reverse.[1]

—**Kris Carr**, cancer survivor turned wellness activist
and author of the *New York Times* bestseller *Crazy Sexy Diet:*
Eat Your Veggies, Ignite Your Spark, and Live Like You Mean It!

As you begin the adventurous Bounce Back Boldly Plan, your first activity is to Nudge Yourself to Eat Better. To understand what I mean, we'll look at a fascinating area of behavioral psychology known as *nudge theory.*

A nudge "alters people's behavior in a predictable way without forbidding any options," behavioral economist and Nobel Prize winner Richard H. Thaler, PhD, and Cass Sunstein explain in their books, *Nudge: Improving Decisions About Health, Wealth, and Happiness*, and *Nudge: The Final Edition.*[2]

If you spend time around man's best friend, you know how effective a nudge can be. When you eat around your pooch, your buddy may gently lay his/her head on your lap and look up at you longingly with those soft, sweet eyes. Of course, at that point, you're a goner. You'll give your doggy a treat.

If, on the other hand, your pet barks loudly, incessantly scampers around while pawing on your belongings, or sneakily snatches food off the table, you'll likely give your canine a time out.

Don't reward yourself with food.
You are not a dog.[3]
—Anonymous

What does this discussion about adorable dogs have to do with you and your plan to peel off pounds?

Whether you realize it or not, you're likely on the receiving end of many nudges daily.

The fact that tempting cookies, crackers, or chips are displayed at eye level in the supermarket? That's a *nudge.* Your waiter reciting the dessert of the day? Another *nudge.* Being asked if you want to supersize that? Again, a *nudge.*[4]

Nudges entice us, but they *don't force* us to take certain action. Rather, they *grab* our attention and *guide* us toward a specific outcome.[5]

Now that you're familiar with this remarkable tactic—which the food industry has effectively used to entice you with unhealthy junk foods—you'll flip the script.

THE PROOF:
The Fascinating Science about Nudging

Promising research shows that nudging can lead us to make healthier food choices:

- **Nudges led to a 15 percent increase in healthier dietary choices.** Nudging guided people to choose better foods and reduce caloric consumption, according to a study published in *BMC Public Health*.[6]
- **Behavioral nudges encourage healthier eating.** According to an analysis in *Marketing Science*, behavioral nudging is the most effective way to reduce your consumption of unhealthy foods (such as offering healthy food on smaller plates).[7]
- **Empowering self-nudges work well.** You're more successful when you design a healthy "decision environment" (as scientists call it) in your home, office, or car, according to a study in *Behavioural Public Policy*.[8]

FEASTS (Fast, Easy, Awesome, Simple, Tested Strategies) to Set Up Healthy Nudges

Today you'll start some out-of-sight, out-of-mind nudges to make healthy eating at home and work automatic. Here are tips to get going:

- **Ditch all caloric sweeteners and foods containing them.** Clean out your fridge, freezer, and pantry. Then place all cookies, crackers, chips, or other unhealthy food substances in a bag, box, or tote. Look for the following sweeteners:

Sugar's Many Names (Partial List)

Agave	Brown sugar
Barley malt	Cane sugar
Beet juice	Caramel
Brown rice syrup	Coconut sugar

Corn syrup

Date sugar

Dextrose

Evaporated cane juice

Fructose (or other sweeteners ending in -ose)

Fruit juice concentrate

Galactose

Glucose

High fructose corn syrup

Honey

Maple syrup

Maltose

Molasses

Raw sugar

Rice syrup

Sorghum syrup

Sucrose[9]

- **Toss artificial sweeteners**. Now take all sweet additives manufactured in labs and add them to your piles of refined foods to discard. Look for:

Saccharin (Sweet'N Low)

Acesulfame potassium (Sweet One)

Aspartame (Equal or NutraSweet)

Neotame (Newtame)

Sucralose (Splenda)

Cyclamate (Banned in the United States but sold in 100+ countries)[10]

- **Get all junk foods out of sight.** Remove all processed foods from your home. Many people like to donate everything to a food bank.[11] If your spouse or partner objects to your ditching their favorite junk foods, come up with a workable compromise. Ask them to join you for all three weeks of the Bounce Back Diet. If they can't or won't, ask them to please eat junk foods outside the home. (Please note that this diet is for adults only, because children and adolescents have different nutritional needs, but you still don't want to keep junk foods in the house.)

You can disrupt a behavior you don't want by removing the prompt. This isn't always easy, but removing the prompt is your best first move to stop a behavior from happening.[12]

—**BJ Fogg, PhD**, behavior scientist at Stanford University and author of the *New York Times* bestseller, *Tiny Habits: The Small Changes That Change Everything*

Buy Groceries and Set Up
More Healthy Home Nudges

Now, if you haven't done so yet, go grocery shopping:

- **Learn what foods to buy.** Before each week of the Bounce Back Diet in Part IV, you'll find shopping lists and meal plans. Purchase foods for the first seven days. See pages 227 to 250.
- **Choose where to shop.** Go to pages 231 to 233 to find links to grocery stores, farmers' markets, and delivery services.
- **Stay in the healthy aisles.** If you go to a supermarket, shop in the store's outer perimeters where you'll find vegetables, fruits, meats, and eggs. Avoid sections containing junk foods. If you shop online, click only links to ingredients on your shopping list.

Once you've filled your fridge, here are more nudges that gently coax you to make healthy eating automatic:

- **Prep healthy nibbles.** Chop up some low-carb, low-calorie vegetables such as celery, cucumbers, lettuce, broccoli, or red pepper slices. Store them in your fridge.
- **Freeze berries.** Measure half-cup portions of fresh or frozen berries, place them in reusable, metal containers, and put in the freezer. (This is one of my favorite portion-control nudges.)
- **Get smaller dishes.** Invest in plates and/or bowls that are one half or a third the size of those you now use. Or eat from lunch, salad, or dessert plates. Research in the *Journal of the Association for Consumer Research* suggests that, on average, halving your plate size led to a 30 percent reduction of the food consumed.[13]
- **Create drink-water nudges.** Take one or two pitchers, measure how many eight-ounce portions they contain, and keep refilling them with water. (To find out how much water you need, take half your body weight in ounces. Learn more on Day 9, *Enjoy Water's Wonders.*)
- **Keep track.** Start a journal to stay motivated daily, monitor your progress, and stay focused on your dreams and goals.

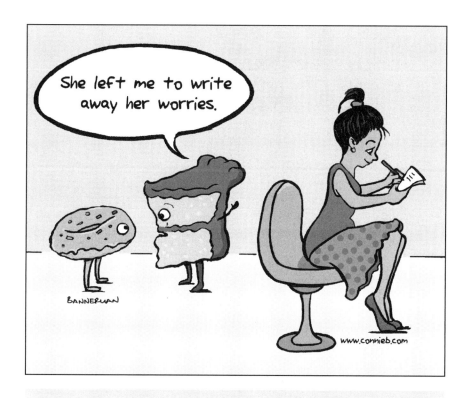

Beyond-the-Book Support:
Get Your Sample of
The Bounce Back Diet Journal

To motivate you daily, I created *The Bounce Back Diet Journal*, which gives you space to write down your goals and affirmations, keep gratitude lists, track your workouts and visualizations, read inspiring quotes, and jot down insights. To find out how to get three weeks of *The Bounce Back Diet Journal*, go to www.BounceBackDiet.com/Book-Bonuses.

DAY 2

DITCH YOUR WHAT-THE-HELL ATTITUDE, CLAIM A CAN-CONTROL OUTLOOK, AND LET GOALPOWERPLUS GUIDE YOU

*If you have the courage to start,
you have the courage to succeed.*[1]

—**Mel Robbins**, motivational expert and *New York Times*
bestselling author of *The 5 Second Rule* and *The High 5 Habit*

You're now ready to toss toxic thoughts, which are the enemies of weight loss. Today you'll Ditch Your *What-the-Hell Attitude*, which can drag you down and derail your weight loss efforts.

Let me explain: Recall a time you were avoiding fattening foods, skipping late-night snacks, and enjoying your healthier body. Then one day you felt stressed out, upset, or anxious, and junk foods beckoned. You took a few bites.

Suddenly, three words came bubbling to the surface and drowned out all others. "What the hell," you thought. "Since I blew my diet, I might as well have [name your big trigger foods]."

You know what came next. You caved in, chewing and chomping into oblivion. Then you couldn't stop.

Overeating quickly became your new norm. Still, you kept promising yourself: "I'll start a new diet tomorrow." But that day still hasn't come.

Right after your binge(s), you felt dejected, discouraged, and disappointed with yourself. You felt overcome by blame and shame. Now you've gotten stuck in a dismal place I call the *What-the-Hell Swampland*.

*"The obstacle in the path becomes the path. Never forget, within
every obstacle is an opportunity to improve our condition."*[2]

—**Ryan Holiday**, bestselling author of *The Obstacle Is the
Way: The Timeless Art of Turning Trials into Triumph*

Researchers Identified This Dangerous *What-the-Hell Effect*

What-the-Hell behavior is so pervasive among dieters that scientists have studied it. They may call it counter-regulation, but we'll just call it the What-the-Hell effect.

This phenomenon reflects the dieter's "mere belief that he [or she] has overeaten is sufficient to trigger an eating binge," explained University of Toronto researcher Janet Polivy, PhD, who is credited with coining the "What-the-Hell" phrase in the 1970s with her colleague C. Peter Herman, PhD.[3]

In short, once you feel that you blew your diet, you keep pigging out on more unhealthy foods and are sucked into a cycle of indulgence and regret.

"It's not the first giving-in that guarantees the bigger relapse," health psychologist Kelly McGonigal, PhD, explains in her book *The Willpower Instinct: How Self-Control Works, Why It Matters, and What You Can Do to Get More of It*.[4]

"It's the feelings of shame, guilt, loss of control and loss of hope that follow the first relapse," she adds.

By the way, researchers found that the What-the-Hell phenomenon also can get the upper hand over other counter-productive habits such as smoking two packs of cigarettes a day, excessive drinking, compulsive shopping, frequent gambling, and endless doom scrolling.[5]

*Be very careful what you say to yourself because
someone very important is listening . . . YOU!*[6]

—**John Assaraf**, entrepreneur, founder/CEO of MyNeuroGym,
and author of the *New York Times* bestselling book *Having It All*

THE PROOF: The Fascinating Science about the *What-the-Hell Effect*

Let's now look at what can happen when you dwell in self-defeatist What-the-Hell behavior and negative self-talk:

- **People eat more cookies if they think that they've already eaten too many.** First, let's turn to a famous pizza-and-cookies experiment from University of Toronto scientists Dr. Polivy and Dr. Herman. For their study, which was published in *Appetite*, the investigators served a slice of pizza to hungry participants, who were asked to taste and rate some cookies. Although everyone received the *exact same size* slice of pizza, some participants received a piece that *looked* larger. Although they believed that they'd eaten *more* than the other participants, they actually consumed the same amount. The result? When *nondieters* wrongly believed that they'd eaten a *bigger* slice, they ate *fewer* cookies to compensate for the calories. But when *dieters* were convinced that they'd eaten a *bigger* slice, they ate *more* cookies. That's the What-the-Hell effect in action.[7]

- **Those who downplay the importance of their goals give up more easily.** When 1,300-plus participants were told that they'd failed a cognitive or academic test, they downplayed how good they'd feel if they succeeded, according to a review in the *Journal of Experimental Social Psychology*. Those subjects who were *strongly motivated to succeed* weren't impacted. Their motivation surpassed everything. The researchers called this tendency to underestimate their desire to achieve their goals *the sour-grape effect* because they considered them unattainable. (The name comes from the *Aesop's* fable, "The Fox and the Grapes.")[8]

- **Overweight women criticize themselves and their weight.** A survey of more than 2,200 women in a community-based weight management program in the United Kingdom found that self-criticism was significantly associated with decreased well-being and higher BMI. The findings, which were published in *PLOS One*, also revealed that females who used self-reassuring strategies and positive social comparisons were more successful at shedding pounds and felt better about their weight.[9]

- **Negative emotions lead people with type 2 diabetes to make poor dietary choices.** Other investigators found that people with type 2 diabetes who fell off their doctor-recommended diets felt frustrated, depressed, angry, and guilty. Those harmful emotions paved the way to more poor dietary choices and negative feelings, according to research in *SAGE Open*. The study's title is revealing: "Wavering Diabetic Diet: 'I Break the Diet and Then I Feel Guilty and Then I Don't Go Back to It, In Case I Feel Guilty Again.'"[10]

Frame your world with your words. . . . Your body is not in control of your mind—your mind is in control of your body, and your mind is stronger than your body. Mind certainly is over matter.[11]

—**Caroline Leaf, PhD**, pathologist, neuroscientist, and bestselling author of *Switch On Your Brain: The Key to Peak Happiness, Thinking, and Health*

MORE PROOF: The Fascinating Science about a *Can-Control Outlook*

Now we'll move on to happier outcomes. You'll learn about adopting an attitude of *perceived control* (as researchers describe it) or a *Can-Control Outlook* as I refer to it. Let's look at scientific findings, which show this at work:

- **Believing that you're in control helps you maintain weight loss.** For a study published in *Behaviour Research and Therapy*, researchers looked at nearly 250 men and women who'd previously lost at least 10 percent of their body weight. Those who successfully kept off the weight were *much more likely* to believe that they were *in charge* of events in their life. On the other hand, people who regained the weight they'd shed were more likely to believe that they exercised little control.[12]

- **When you think you're in command, you can positively affect outcomes.** For a *Frontiers in Neuroscience* study, scientists suggested that individuals who felt out of control were more likely to feel depressed and anxious and have a greater chance of succumbing to a downward spiral. However, those who perceived *they were in control* over events or situations had improved mental and physical health. This empowering attitude, the researchers speculated, "is a strong predictor of achievement in life."[13]

- **When you focus on growth, you see setbacks as part of the learning process.** Now we come to one of my favorite conclusions. When you're sufficiently motivated to change, you can persist and persevere despite any challenges. Indeed, "growth-minded individuals perceive task setbacks as a necessary part of the learning process and they 'bounce back' by increasing their motivational effort," research scientist Betsy Ng, PhD, wrote in a review paper about growth mindset and intrinsic motivation in the publication *Brain Sciences*.[14]

The passion for stretching yourself and sticking to it, even (or especially) when it's not going well, is the hallmark of the growth mindset.[15]

—**Carol S. Dweck, PhD**, psychologist, researcher, Stanford University professor, and author of *Mindset: The New Psychology of Success*

Additional Proof: Visualizations And Affirmations

We have two more concepts to explore—the amazing results of repeating affirmations and doing visualizations. Let's look at some compelling evidence-based findings:

- **Mental imagery helps you eat better when you add implementation intentions.** Psychologists showed that you can use the sports psychology technique of doing vivid and detailed mental rehearsals and apply it to eating better by adding *implementation intentions*. These are "if-then" plans that specify when, where, and how you'll carry out a goal or react if you encounter any challenges. (You'd prepare by thinking, "If I encounter situation Y, then I'll do this [goal-directed] behavior Z.") For the study, published in *Psychology and Health*, more than 230 students set a goal of eating more fruit for a week. Those who made an action plan and visualized achieving the goal consumed twice as much fruit as those who just set the goal. "Telling people to just change the way they eat doesn't work. But research shows that if people make a concrete plan about what they are going to do, they are better at acting on their intentions," explained McGill University health psychology professor Bärbel Knäuper, PhD, who spearheaded the study. "What we've done that's new is to add visualization techniques to the action plan," she clarified to me.[16]

- **Affirmations light up our brains.** Scientists writing in *Social Cognitive and Affective Neuroscience* used functional magnetic resonance imaging (fMRI) to explore whether self-affirmation statements activate areas of the brain involved in expecting and receiving reward. Participants were asked to rank their top core values. Then they lay in a brain scanner and thought (as advised) about a scenario involving a top core value. "When affirmed individuals (compared to unaffirmed) contemplated something near and dear to their hearts, their brains' reward centers lit up like beautifully decorated Christmas trees," the study's lead author Christopher Cascio, PhD, clarified. Now get this: The brain scans showed that the areas in the brain activated by affirmations are *the same reward centers* that respond to other pleasurable experiences, such as eating your favorite meal or winning a prize. "Affirmation takes advantage of our reward circuits, which can be quite powerful," added Dr. Cascio, an assistant professor at the University of Wisconsin's School of Journalism and Mass Communication.[17]

▪ **Repeating affirmations may help you shed weight.** Scientists writing in *Psychological Science* found that after two-and-a-half months, self-affirming women weighed less, had lower BMIs, and had smaller waistlines than those who didn't do affirmations.[18]

Bounce Back Boldly Weight Success Story

My diet wasn't clean at all. I was really frustrated and sick and tired of not achieving my fitness goals. One day I heard a speaker on a podcast say, "If you want radical results, you should make radical changes."

I cut out sugar, wheat, dairy, gluten, alcohol, and coffee and I saw radical results. Every morning, I read my vision statement. I would visualize often. And I repeated an affirmation several times a day. I would say, "I am 175 pounds, fit, healthy, flexible, vibrant, and full of energy."[19]

—**Mat Boggs**, relationship expert, bestselling author, cofounder of the Brave Thinking Institute, and YouTuber, who shed and has kept off twenty-five pounds for five years and running.

Compelling Proof About
Setting and Achieving Goals

Keep your eyes on the prize, as the saying goes. When you focus on reachable goals, you'll find it easier, even effortless, to stay on track. Let me introduce you to an amazing trait that I call *GoalPowerPlus*. This is when you continue to unleash your burning desire, which drives you to reach for important goals (your *whys*) so you'll feel better, have energy, and achieve your other dreams. Let's now look at some findings about goal-setting:

- **When you zero in on approach goals, you'll get better results.** Research published in the *American Journal of Lifestyle Medicine* indicates that when you focus on *approach goals* (when, where, and how you'll do something), you'll achieve them more easily because you're moving *toward* a desired outcome. On the one hand, *avoidance goals* (what you don't want) are linked to "fewer positive thoughts and greater negative emotions." On the other hand, approach goals are associated with positive emotions. ("If I eat a healthy dinner tonight, I'll feel better, and then I'll be on track to reaching my target weight.")[20]
- **If you write down your goals, you have greater success.** Subjects who put their goals in writing were 33 percent more successful than those who didn't, according to research from Gail Matthews, PhD, an adjunct psychology professor at Dominican University of California. In addition, more than 70 percent of participants who sent weekly updates to a friend were more successful at achieving their goals than 35 percent of those who kept their goals to themselves and didn't write them down.[21]
- **It's easier to achieve goals when you make the process fun.** You'll stand a better chance of reaching your goals when you pair "a pleasurable indulgence with a behavior that provides delayed rewards," explains Katy Milkman, PhD, a professor at the Wharton School at the University of Pennsylvania, and author of the *New York Times* bestseller *How to Change: The Science of Getting from Where You Are to Where You Want to Be.*[22] Dr. Milkman calls this *temptation bundling.* Here's how to do it: You "bundle" a source of instant gratification like watching a TV show with a less fun, "should" activity like working out. In fact, for one of Dr. Milk-

man's studies, the researchers gave subjects iPods loaded with audiobooks, but they could listen *only* while working out at the gym. After four weeks, they boosted their likelihood of working out by 10 to 14 percent, according to their research published in *Organizational Behavior and Human Decision Processes*.[23]

> *Research has proven time and again that rather than relying on willpower to resist temptation, we're better off figuring out how to make good behaviors more gratifying in the short-term.*[24]

—**Katy Milkman, PhD**, behavioral scientist and author of *How to Change*

FEASTS (Fast, Easy, Awesome, Simple, Tested Strategies) to Claim a *Can-Control Outlook* and Choose *GoalPowerPlus*

You've learned about some powerful, proven practices that pave the way to success. Now you'll put the fascinating findings to use:

- **Claim a Can-Control Outlook.** Every day, step into a powerful, positive, proactive attitude. Own your complete control. Step into that awesome unstoppable feeling. Choose empowering words. Speak to yourself as if you're your bestie.
- **Go for GoalPowerPlus.** Be specific. Write down your goals. How many pounds do you want to shed? What indoor or outdoor activities do you enjoy? What will be your exercise routine? What other big goals do you have? Journal about these topics.[25]
- **Turn your goals into affirmations and ramp up your desire to reach them.** Create affirmations that clarify your goals, and state them aloud enthusiastically every morning, afternoon, and evening. (For instance: *I am enjoying walking two miles a day, and I am in great health.*)
- **Develop fun routines to reach your goals.** Use temptation bundling while you move towards your desired weight. For instance, watch a TED talk or repeat affirmations while you walk in place at home.
- **Applaud and encourage yourself in the third person.** Give yourself pep talks while you refer to yourself by your first name. Research from the *Journal of Personality and Social Psychology* suggests

that "small shifts in the language people use to refer [to them-selves can] consequentially influence their ability to regulate their thoughts, feelings, and behavior."[26]

- **Keep doing the DDEVA steps.** To refresh your memory, you want to feel your DESIRE for better health; DECIDE to achieve your goals; EXPECT success; VISUALIZE your awesome body; and AFFIRM often that you'll be triumphant.
- **Continue to confidently proclaim your favorite Bounce Back Boldly affirmations.**

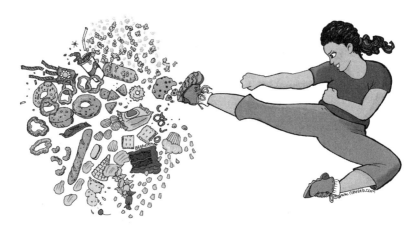

You can kick culprit carbs!

Beyond-the-Book Support: Get Help to Activate *GoalPowerPlus*

Let me guide you to zero in on your goals. Get help to activate GoalPowerPlus at www.BounceBackDiet.com/Book-Bonuses.

DAY 3

BEGIN THE DAY WITH A BALANCED BREAKFAST

One of the most important things you can do for your health is to avoid a breakfast that is sweet (made of just sugar and starch, like oats with fruit puree). This helps reduce inflammation and cravings for the rest of the day.[1]

—**Jessie Inchauspé**, aka Glucose Goddess, biochemist,
and author of the *Glucose Revolution:
The Life-Changing Power of Balancing Your Blood Sugar*

It's time to stop neglecting that important first meal of the day.

Too many people treat breakfast as an afterthought while running out the door. In fact, nearly one-fifth of Americans skip the morning meal, and the rest load up on carbs and coffee.[2]

That's too bad. Research shows that regularly giving breakfast the cold shoulder may increase your odds of gaining weight.[3] What's more, not eating in the morning may raise your risk of such health problems as heart disease, high blood pressure, high cholesterol, and memory impairment.[4] On the other hand, having breakfast every a.m. may kickstart your metabolism, boost your brainpower, balance blood sugar levels, improve your moods, and make you more physically active.[5]

THE PROOF:
The Fascinating Science about a Balanced Breakfast

Breakfast is unique among meals, because you're breaking a fast. Assuming that you didn't snack after dinner or grab a midnight snack, your body hasn't taken in any nutrients for eight or more hours. Trying to start your day without eating is like trying to turn on your car without gas. Consider:

- **Ignoring the morning meal may increase the risk of obesity by nearly 50 percent.** Scientists reviewed 45 observational studies and found that those who ate nothing between 5 a.m. and 9 a.m. or consumed only sweets such as pastries or cookies during that time increased their risk of being overweight or obese by 48 percent. Skipping breakfast also increased the risk of abdominal obesity by 31 percent, the researchers pointed out in *Obesity Research and Clinical Practice*.[6] (Abdominal obesity is extra fat around the midsection associated with an increased risk for many health problems, including: type 2 diabetes, cancer, cardiovascular disease, hypertension, and metabolic syndrome.)[7]

- **Eating more at breakfast leads to greater weight loss and other health benefits.** For three months, overweight women focused on eating more at breakfast (700 kcal for breakfast, 500 kcal at lunch, and 200 kcal come dinner) or the reverse (200 kcal at breakfast, 500 kcal at lunch, and 700 kcal at dinner). The study, which was published in the journal *Obesity*, revealed that those who ate larger breakfasts had greater weight loss and waist circumference reduction. They also experienced a significant decrease in fasting glucose and insulin levels and had a 33.6 percent decrease in triglyceride levels.[8]

Indeed, research shows that eating breakfast makes it easier to shed and keep off extra pounds. Let's look at one more study:

- **Eating in the morning helps burn more calories.** In an experiment published in *The Journal of Clinical Endocrinology & Metabolism*, researchers gave men of a healthy body weight either a big-breakfast-and-small-dinner combo or the opposite. All subjects took in the same number of calories, but on mornings when they ate a large breakfast, they burned two-and-a-half times more calories than on days when they had a bigger dinner. [9]

The Pluses of a Well-Rounded PFF Breakfast —and all Meals

Good things often come in threes. Take, for example, a winning row of tic-tac-toe, "The Three Little Pigs" of fable fame, and now, your secret weight loss arsenal. PFF is my shorthand for Protein, Fiber, and (high quality) Fat. Taking in ample PFF fills you up and makes it easier to shed pounds without feeling deprived.

- **P: Protein** is satiating, which means you feel full longer. Protein, which is digested slowly, plays a key role in metabolism by preserving muscle, your body's most metabolically active tissue.[10] Studies show that protein reduces appetite, increases fat burning, and helps maintain weight loss. [11]

- **F: Fiber**, both the soluble and insoluble kind, has been linked to numerous health benefits, but the average American gets only sixteen grams a day of this beneficial nutrient.[12] To shed weight, you want to consume at least thirty grams of fiber a day, according to a study in the *Annals of Internal Medicine*.[13]
- **F: Fat** still makes people nervous. But you need healthy monounsaturated and polyunsaturated fats (MUFAs and PUFAs), which are found in avocadoes, olive oil, olives, nuts, chia seeds, and fatty fish such as salmon, trout, and mackerel. Like protein, healthy fats are digested slowly and are satiating.[14]

Eating well-rounded, PFF-filled, blood-sugar-balanced breakfasts isn't enough. All meals and snacks should keep your blood sugar levels steady. A study in *Nature Metabolism* found that people experiencing big drops in their blood sugar levels several hours after eating ended up feeling hungrier and consuming hundreds more calories during the day.[15] While you follow the Bounce Back Diet, you'll eat balanced meals at suggested intervals, which will keep your blood sugar levels stable.

FEASTS (Fast, Easy, Awesome, Simple, Tested Strategies) to Eat Breakfast

Here are some ways to streamline your morning eating routine:

- **Carve out time.** To make your morning sail smoothly, set your alarm fifteen to thirty minutes earlier so you can have time for your first meal of the day.
- **Make morning the time you step into a positive attitude for the day.** As you prepare your and/or your family's nutritious breakfast, repeat positive affirmations. While you eat, visualize those quality foods making you healthier.
- **Prep the night before.** Cut up vegetables, wash or freeze fruit, or hard-boil eggs in advance.
- **Eat leftovers.** Switch up your breakfast. The morning after a healthy dinner, eat leftover veggies and a modest portion of meat or fish from the night before. (You'll do this several times on the Bounce Back Diet.)

Now you know about the tremendous power of eating healthy PFF foods the first thing every morning. Let your balanced breakfasts get your days off to a stupendous start.

DAY 4

FREE YOURSELF FROM THE MONKEY MIND

I am burdened with what the Buddhists call the monkey mind.
The thoughts that swing from limb to limb, stopping only to
scratch themselves, spit and howl. My mind swings wildly through time,
touching on dozens of ideas a minute, unharnessed and undisciplined.[1]

—**Elizabeth Gilbert,** journalist and #1 *New York Times*
bestselling author of *Eat, Pray, Love*

Nearly 3,000 years ago, the Buddha reportedly observed that when he felt overwhelmed by thoughts, he felt as though monkeys were inside his brain, chattering and jumping from branch to branch.[2]

You may feel similarly. Like noisy monkeys bouncing from branch to branch, your worries, ideas, and to-do list can gang up on you and leave you feeling anxious, overwhelmed, or easily rattled.

Not only that, but your *monkey mind* also can make it difficult to lose weight. This is why you want to learn to claim calm.

Perhaps the best way to quiet your monkey mind is to meditate.

THE PROOF: The Fascinating Science about Mindfulness Meditation

Although you can choose from a variety of ways to meditate, we'll zero in on easy-to-learn mindfulness meditation.[3] This is when you pay attention to the natural rhythm and flow of your breaths as well as to any feelings, thoughts, or sensations when they arise.

Mindfulness meditation intentionally cultivates "nonjudgmental moment-to-moment awareness," explains Jon Kabat-Zinn, PhD, founder of the acclaimed Mindfulness-Based Stress Reduction Clinic (MBSR) at the University of Massachusetts Medical School.[4]

A large body of research has found that with regular practice, mindfulness meditation may reduce anxiety, improve focus, lessen emotional reactivity, boost immune functioning, decrease fatigue, improve sleep, help with pain management, increase self-awareness, mitigate cognitive decline, and make you more positive.[5]

Mindfulness meditation also can help you cut back on bingeing, shed weight, and triumph over eating disorders. For instance:

- **Mindfulness meditators may eat less and choose healthier foods.** Researchers found that obese subjects who practiced mindfulness meditation shed an average of fifteen pounds over six months as opposed to nonmeditators, who lost nine pounds. Those who meditated also found it easier to stick to eating healthier foods and refrain from overeating, according to the study in the *Journal of Complementary and Integrative Medicine.*[6]

- **People who practice mindfulness meditation may binge less.** Similarly, a review of studies, published in *Eating Behaviors,* concluded that "mindfulness meditation effectively decreases binge eating and emotional eating in populations engaging in this behavior."[7]

- **Meditators shed belly fat.** A study in the *Journal of Obesity* found that women who received four months of mindfulness meditation training managed stress better and lost more deep abdominal fat than nonmeditators.[8] They also demonstrated significant reductions in their cortisol awakening response, or CAR. (This is a diagnostic marker of stress that measures how much cortisol is in the blood within an hour of waking.)

When you learn to navigate and manage your breath,
you can navigate any situation in life.[9]

—**Jay Shetty**, former monk, purpose coach, and author of the #1 *New York Times* bestseller *Think Like a Monk*

FEASTS (Fast, Easy, Awesome, Simple, Tested Strategies) to Practice Mindfulness Meditation

Here are some tips to make mindfulness meditation a part of your everyday life:

- **Make it a daily routine.** Meditate at the same time very day. For instance, I meditate the first thing every morning.

- **Even a few minutes help.** You can experience better moods, enhanced attentiveness, and decreased anxiety by meditating as little as thirteen minutes a day, according to a study published in *Behavioural Brain Research*.[10]

- **You can meditate almost anywhere.** You don't need a meditation room or space. You can meditate on a plane, train, bus, or in an office cubicle.
- **Here are steps to get started with mindfulness meditation**.
  1. Find a quiet place to sit on a chair or cross-legged on the floor. If you prefer, lie down so your spine is straight, but don't go to sleep.
  2. Close your eyes.
  3. Notice your natural breathing without trying to change it.
  4. Feel your breaths go in and out.
  5. Let your thoughts come and go without judgment.
  6. When your mind begins to wander, just gently and non-judgmentally bring it back to your breath.[11]

Today you learned an important habit. By starting to focus on your breath, you've laid a valuable foundation to lead a calmer, happier life.

Beyond-the-Book Support:
Mindfulness Meditation Resources

To get links to some free mindfulness meditation resources, see my blog post at www.connieb.com/Mindfulness-Meditation-Resources.

DAY 5

DRINK BONE BROTH OR CHICKEN SOUP

Bone broth isn't just broth. And it isn't just soup. It's concentrated healing. This broth is nutrient-rich "liquid gold," one of the world's oldest and most powerful medicinal foods.[1]

—**Kellyann Petrucci, ND,** naturopathic physician, certified nutrition consultant, and author of the *New York Times* bestseller *Dr. Kellyann's Bone Broth Diet*

For thousands of years, nutrient-rich bone broth has been a staple in cultures around the world.[2]

This tasty yellow or golden drink—which is made by simmering animal bones in water until the bones give up their nutrients, collagen, and flavor—has gained a following among ketogenic and Paleo devotees, competitive athletes, people seeking to resolve health issues, and health enthusiasts.[3]

Fans of this much-touted elixir also reportedly include celebrities such as Halle Berry, Salma Hayek, Gwyneth Paltrow, Mindy Kaling, Goldie Hawn, Ryan Seacrest, and Shailene Woodley.[4]

Most devotees of bone broth agree that this low-calorie beverage helps stave off hunger and fills you up.[5] Its culinary relative, chicken soup (without gluten-filled noodles), also helps curb appetite.[6]

If you drink one or more cups a day of homemade or superior-sourced, low-calorie bone broth or chicken soup in the late morning, mid-afternoon, or before dinner, you'll find it easier to avoid unhealthy snacks.

I count quality bone broth as an important supplemental food. The copious health benefits are simply too substantial to pass up.[7]

—**Mark Sisson**, founder of www.marksdailyapple.com and Primal Kitchen

THE PROOF: The Fascinating Science about Bone Broth and Chicken Soup

Bone broth has long been thought to have medicinal properties. Back in the Stone Age 2.6 million years ago, our prehistoric ancestors were "cooking broth in turtle shells and in skins over the fire," Sally Fallon Morell and Kaayla Daniel, PhD, wrote in their book *Nourishing Broth: An Old-Fashioned Remedy for a Modern World.*[8]

In the 5th century BC, Hippocrates, "the father of medicine," advised people with digestive issues to drink bone broth.[9] Later, in the 12th century AD, the medieval rabbi, philosopher, and physician Maimonides recommended the "Jewish penicillin" for asthma and weight gain.[10]

Nowadays, this beverage is popular around the world. In Italy, it's called *brodo*; in France, it's *bouillon*; and in Portugal and Spain, it's *caldo.*[11]

The benefits of bone broth are still being studied, but advocates maintain that this liquid gold may boost weight loss, curtail cravings, strengthen bones, improve joint health, alleviate allergies or food intolerances, boost the immune system, reduce inflammation, and aid sleep.[12]

Here are a few highlights from research about bone broth or chicken soup:

- **People who drink bone broth may consume fewer calories.** Research published in *Appetite* observed that after drinking a chicken broth-based soup before a meal, subjects consumed 20 percent fewer calories overall compared to people who didn't have any soup.[13]

- **Bone broth has anti-inflammatory properties.** A study in the publication, *Medicina,* showed that due to the anti-inflammatory benefits, consuming bone broth may decrease symptoms of ulcerative colitis.[14]

- **Chicken soup has medicinal qualities.** A study from the journal *Chest* noticed that eating chicken soup enhanced the activity of neutrophils, white blood cells that fight infections and help heal damaged tissue.[15]

- **Eating soup helps people keep off the weight.** A review of seven different studies published in *Physiology and Behavior* found that those who consumed soup were 15 percent less likely to be obese.[16]

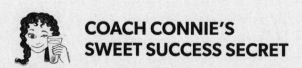

COACH CONNIE'S SWEET SUCCESS SECRET

Bone Broth Keeps My Blood Sugar Levels Stable

Bone broth is one of my favorite beverages. For instance, I usually enjoy a cup before breakfast so I don't get too hungry during my hour-long, empowering morning routine. In addition, I may sip bone broth in the late afternoon.

What I love about bone broth is that it helps to balance my blood sugar levels, fills me up, keeps me from unnecessary snacking, has few calories, and is quite tasty.

FEASTS (Fast, Easy, Awesome, Simple, Tested Strategies) to Enjoy Bone Broth or Chicken Soup

Here are some tips to make the most out of your new beverage habit:

- **Try bone broth or chicken soup with or without veggies as a low-calorie, low-carb snack.** This beverage makes a quick post-workout snack, mid-afternoon pick-me-up, or before-dinner beverage.
- **Add bone broth to sauces, soups, stews, and eggs.** Whenever you cook vegetables, omelets, sauces, or stews, use bone broth or chicken soup as the liquid to give your dishes more nutrients and flavor.
- **Make your own.** To make bone broth from scratch, see recipe on page 270.

Here's wishing you a savory exploration into the world of healthy, low-calorie bone broth. Once you start sipping, you'll find, I predict, that it gives you energy, tastes yummy, and satisfies your appetite.

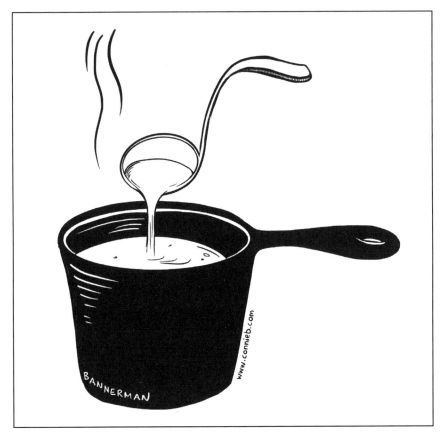

"Yum! Bone broth is so tasty, filling, and nourishing."

Beyond-the-Book Support:
Resources for Premade Bone Broth

To order frozen or powdered bone broth, see a selected list of vendors on my blog at www.connieb.com/where-to-buy-quality-bone-broth.

DAY 6

TAP AWAY YOUR CRAVINGS, STRESS, OR GRIEF

What tapping does, with amazing efficiency, is halt the fight-or-flight response and . . . send a calming response to the body. . . . More than ever, we need tools like this to find peace, to find balance.[1]

—**Nick Ortner**, founder of the Tapping World Summit, creator and executive producer of *The Tapping Solution* film, and author of the *New York Times* bestseller *The Tapping Solution: A Revolutionary System for Stress-Free Living*

Today, I'm excited to tell you about an easy, powerful, scientifically validated technique that can help you shut down cravings for junk foods, decrease anxiety, dial down depression, reduce insomnia, improve physical pain, calm your performance jitters, and much more.

Emotional Freedom Technique, or EFT—better known as tapping—is one of the easiest, fastest, most effective tools you'll use to triumph over troubling situations, squash your cravings, or quickly calm down.

What's so great about tapping is that you can do it on and by yourself at any time whenever you seek relief.

How EFT (Tapping) Works

Rooted in the 3,000-year-old technique of acupuncture, EFT was developed in the late 1990s by neurolinguistic practitioner Gary Craig to alleviate anxiety.[2]

Tapping combines Eastern medicine and Western psychology.[3] It is based on the premise from Chinese medicine that all negative emotions can be traced to a disruption in the body's energy system.

With EFT, all you do is lightly tap with your fingertips on nine meridian energy points through which body energy flows, while you focus on any negative emotions and make certain statements.[4] This process restores balance to your disrupted energy.

Tapping does this by targeting the amygdala, the part of the brain that fires off the stress response to help you deal with a real or perceived threat.[5]

Just think of EFT as an easy way to press a reset button which brings you back into balance.

Tapping Has Become More Mainstream

In recent years, EFT has been widely popularized, thanks to EFT experts and siblings Nick, Jessica, and Alex Ortner, who, since 2009, have presented the Tapping World Summit, an annual worldwide online event.[6]

Nowadays, many top experts, bestselling authors, and motivational teachers laud tapping's numerous benefits. For instance, EFT's many advocates include Dr. Mark Hyman, Jack Canfield, Gabrielle Bernstein, Kris Carr, Cheryl Richardson, Tony Robbins, Dr. Kim D'Eramo, Margaret M. Lynch, and Dr. Bessel Van Der Kolk.[7]

Tapping clears cravings, releases frustration about relapses and plateaus, transforms stress reactions that make people overeat, and eliminates the emotional "need" for wearing protection [extra weight] around your body.[8]

—**Carol Look,** EFT Master, psychotherapist,
and author of *Attracting Abundance with EFT*

THE PROOF:
The Fascinating Science about Tapping

To date, more than 130 peer-reviewed clinical trials validate the effectiveness of EFT. For instance, a review in the *Journal of Psychotherapy Integration* found that tapping is "not only effective, but unusually rapid and improvements are durable."[9]

To better understand EFT's increasing use and influence, I reached out to the author of that paper, clinical psychologist David Feinstein, PhD, a recognized leader in the emerging field of energy psychology, which has been described as "acupressure for the emotions."[10]

"As strange as tapping looks, it can quickly and noninvasively alter brain chemistry for therapeutic gain," Dr. Feinstein explained.[11]

Due to the extensive research "supporting its effectiveness, therapists are taking note," Dr. Feinstein added, referring to the fact that the American Psychological Association (APA) offers continuing education accreditation for training in Emotional Freedom Technique.[12]

Let's look at some studies that point to tapping's many benefits:

- **Tapping lowered anxiety, reduced depression, diminished pain, boosted happiness, and much more.** For one investigation of EFT in the *Journal of Evidence-Based Integrative Medicine*, researchers examined thirty-one studies and observed nearly 17,000 people. They found that tapping produced the following changes: immunoglobulin-A (IgA, an antibody blood protein that's part of your immune system) soared by 113 percent; food cravings were reduced by 74 percent; pain went down 57 percent; anxiety dropped 40 percent; cortisol was lessened 37 percent; depression decreased 35 percent; PTSD symptoms were reduced 32 percent; happiness was boosted 31 percent; and resting heart rate went down 8 percent.[13]

- **EFT helped with psychological, physiological, and performance issues.** Another comprehensive research paper, which was published in the peer-reviewed publication *Frontiers in Psychology,* concluded that EFT was effective for psychological conditions such as anxiety, depression, phobias, and PTSD; physiological issues such as pain, insomnia, and autoimmune conditions; professional and sports performance; and biological markers of stress. The study also observed that "few treatment sessions are required, treatment is effective whether delivered in person or virtually, and symptom improvements persist over time."[14]

- **EFT reduced symptoms of PTSD.** Research demonstrated that tapping was an effective, evidence-based treatment for PTSD, according to findings in another study in *Frontiers in Psychology.*[15]

Anxiety loses its grip when tapping enters the scene. Tapping clears the way for you to make healthier choices and diminishes the urge to self-soothe by overeating.[16]

—Mary Ayers, PhD, psychotherapist and coaching specialist, who guides fans to Tap into Action

MORE PROOF: Brain Scans Reveal
That Tapping Can Curb Cravings

Of course, you want to know if tapping can help you dial down your cravings and keep off extra weight.

"EFT is really effective for cravings," says researcher Dawson Church, PhD, founder of the National Institute for Integrative Healthcare, which spearheaded 100 clinical trials about the methodology.[17]

"When people [attend] our workshops, . . . we expose them to the foods they crave" (think chocolate, donuts, bread, and pasta), and the cravings go "down by an average of 83% in just a half hour of tapping," contends Dr. Church, founder of EFT Universe and author of *The Genie in Your Genes.*

Further compelling research about tapping's ability to reduce cravings comes from a team headed by clinical psychologist and EFT researcher Peta Stapleton, PhD, an associate professor at Bond University in Australia and author of *The Science Behind Tapping: A Proven Stress Management Technique for the Mind and Body.*[18]

For a pioneering study published in *OBM Integrative and Complementary Medicine,* Dr. Stapleton and her team took before-and-after brain scans of sugar-craving subjects, who participated in a four-week tapping program. This was the first time functional magnetic resonance imaging [fMRI] was used to "see physical, scientific evidence of exactly how EFT self-help techniques work on these conditions by changing the brain's neural pathways in addiction and food cravings," Dr. Stapleton explained to me via e-mail.[19]

Later, in an eight-week follow-up program that tested EFT's effect on cravings and weight loss, participants also experienced significant changes. "The cravings didn't come back," she amplified.[20]

> *Tapping will work even if you are skeptical.*
> *So try it!*[21]
>
> **—Jack Canfield and Pamela Bruner**,
> authors, *Tapping Into Ultimate Success*

Tapping Points

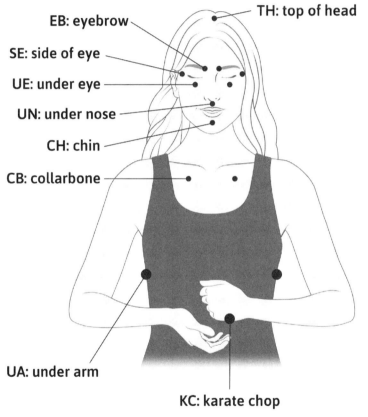

EB: eyebrow

SE: side of eye

UE: under eye

UN: under nose

CH: chin

CB: collarbone

TH: top of head

UA: under arm

KC: karate chop

Reprinted with permission from The Tapping Solution.[22]

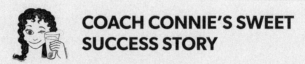

COACH CONNIE'S SWEET SUCCESS STORY

How Tapping Helped Me Cut Out *Carbage*, Heal from Grief, and Now Keeps Me Calm and Productive

When I was plagued by huge carb cravings after losing my mother, I hired an EFT coach to help me quit my dangerous habit. My first assignment was to buy my favorite quickie-carb snacks and bring them to our phone session but not eat a single bite. Talk about unnerving!

For the first few sessions, I was instructed to open packages of movie popcorn, corn nuggets, and sweet potato chips, look at them, inhale their overpowering scents, and even touch the junk foods. All the while, we tapped and I calmly proclaimed, "I love, accept, and approve of myself."

The results were extraordinary. Within several tapping sessions, I *lost all interest* in the quickie carbs that had trapped me for months! Suddenly, I felt powerful, in command, and immune to their temptations. Now, years later, I still easily shun crappy carbs, and my cravings never came back.

Later, I worked with another top tapping expert, who helped me heal from deeper issues such as trauma, betrayal, and abuse. Then we moved on to topics such as staying creative, completing this book, and serving you as best I can.

Nowadays, I still do tapping every day to help me tackle my goals, reduce anxiety, have a productive day, or quiet my busy brain so I can sleep. Every time I do EFT, I continue to be astounded by how well this simple, scientifically validated technique works.

FEASTS (Fast, Easy, Awesome, Simple, Tested Strategies) to do Tapping (EFT)

It's time to discover the wonders of tapping. Here are the easy steps:[23]

- **Notice and name the problem.** Take one to three calming breaths while you identify *exactly* what's going on. What's bugging you? Are you feeling cravings, grief, or anger? The more specific you are, the better. For our purposes, we'll zero in on cravings you have for desserts, quickie carbs, or fast foods.

- **Measure the intensity.** Think about how strong your cravings are for certain trigger foods. Rank the level of your desire for them from 0 to 10. This is called the Subjective Units of Distress, or SUDS, test.

- **Create a setup statement, and then conclude with love, acceptance, and approval for yourself.** Come up with a short sentence that crystalizes the problem you want to eliminate. Gently tap your karate chop point (the fleshy part of the outside of your hand) while you repeat the setup phrase and approval statement three times. Essentially, you want to acknowledge how you feel so you can vanquish it. For example, you could say, "Even though I binged on junk foods when I felt upset [angry, worried, depressed, etc.], I deeply and completely love, accept, and approve of myself."

- **Do two to five rounds of tapping.** Now lightly tap the eight meridian points: eyebrow (EB), side of eyes (SE), under eyes (UE), under nose (UN), under mouth (UM), collarbone (CB), under arms (UA), and top of head (TH) while you say a phrase that reminds you of your setup statement. (See chart on page 147.) Example: "This craving for . . ." or, "This infuriating craving." That's considered one round of tapping.

- **Retake the SUDS test and repeat if needed.** Recheck the level of your cravings, stress, or anxiety. If you're still at a 6, 7, or 8, tap another two or three rounds. Your goal is to reduce your cravings to between 0 and 2 until you feel calm, relieved, and relaxed.

- **End with upbeat statements.** Now that you've recognized your resistance, conclude with two or three rounds of positive programming. Example:
  EB: I can begin to feel good about my body.
  SE: I can begin to feel free.

UE: It's safe for me to take better care of my body.
UN: I'm healthier every day, because I'm eating better every day.
UM: I now imagine my wonderful, active, vibrant future.
CB: I am supported by invisible forces.
UA: It's so easy to eat healthy foods.
TH: Eating healthy is what I do and feeling healthy is who I am!
Take a deep breath in . . . and release it.

Whenever you do this remarkable technique, you can easily address whatever is troubling you, and soon, I predict, you'll feel immense relief.

DISCLAIMER

By sharing information about tapping, I am not dispensing medical advice or prescribing this technique as a form of treatment for physical, emotional, or medical problems. My intent is to offer information to help you in your quest for emotional and spiritual well-being. If you choose to do tapping, the author and publisher assume no responsibility. Although EFT research has found that many people benefit from using tapping for food cravings, weight loss, anxiety, and depression, responses to the technique are individual. This information is not a substitute for traditional medical attention, counseling, therapy, or advice from a qualified health professional.

Beyond-the-Book Support: Get Your Tapping Gift

To help you use EFT to resolve guilt, anger, or shame that you blew your diet, get my complimentary tapping program and companion script. Access it at <u>www.BounceBackDiet.com/Book-Bonuses</u>.

DAY 7

MOVE MORE AND SIT LESS

Physical exercise is the fountain of youth; it's critical to keeping your brain vibrant and young. If you want to attack Alzheimer's disease, depression, obesity, and aging all at once, move every day.[1]

—**Daniel G. Amen**, **MD**, neuroscientist, psychiatrist, brain-imaging expert, head of the Amen Clinics, and *New York Times* bestselling author of *Change Your Brain, Change Your Life*

Perhaps you've heard the saying: "You can't out-exercise a bad diet." That's true. Eating right isn't nearly enough. Movement is essential.

Researchers and health experts agree that you should regularly move your body because you get many physical and mental benefits from exercising.

Don't train to be skinny. Train to be a #badass.[2]

—**Demi Lovato**, singer and songwriter ("I Love Me" and "Confident")

THE PROOF: The Fascinating Science about Exercising and the Weight Loss Connection

Let's look at some health and weight loss benefits of exercise:

- **Physical activity can suppress your appetite.** Researchers found that when participants exercised sixty minutes a day, their risk of overeating dropped by more than half to only 5 percent. Then, for every additional ten minutes of physical activity, the chances of overeating dropped by 1 percent, according to a study in *Health Psychology*.[3]
- **Exercise is more important than diet when it comes to** *maintaining* **weight loss.** For a study published in the journal *Obesity*, University of Colorado researchers following more than 100 adults for four years discovered that weight maintainers burned more calories through regular physical activity and moved more daily, racking up an average of 12,000 steps a day. That's much more than the 9,000 steps taken by normal weight subjects or

6,500 steps by overweight and obese people. Interestingly, all three groups consumed roughly the same number of calories a day.[4]

- **Lifting weights can help you stay trim.** Other scientists who studied the physical activity habits of nearly 12,000 healthy-weight adults aged eighteen to eighty for six years, found that doing both resistance training and aerobic exercise was the best way to prevent obesity. Even without cardio, people who lifted weights at least one hour, two days per week, had a reduced risk of developing obesity, according to the study published in *PLOS Medicine.*[5]

Exercising regularly also has beneficial effects on mood:

- **Working out may treat or prevent anxiety and depression, reduce stress, and boost self-esteem.** You've probably heard about or experienced that coveted "runner's high." That happens because moving your body may trigger the production of *endorphins*, the body's feel-good chemicals and natural painkillers, according to a study published in *Depression and Anxiety.*[6]
- **Walking makes you feel good.** An hour a day of a moderately vigorous activity, such as walking, was linked to a lower risk of depression, according to research published in *JAMA Psychiatry.*[7]

For me, cardio is an essential part of my workout—my fitness regime is not complete without it! [Health] benefits I have experienced include cardio and heart health, improved memory, clear, healthier skin, blood sugar control, reduced fatigue, significant calorie burn, helping maintain a healthy weight, and my personal favorite—increased sexual arousal. So ladies . . . let's go![8]

—**Halle Berry**, Oscar-winning actress inviting her Instagram followers to exercise

PROOF: The Science about "Sitting Disease" and Moving More

Now let's look at the opposite of moving—sitting. Most of us spend a third of our waking hours planted on our rear ends, in large part, because we're at our computers, watching TV or videos, or playing video games.

One in four US adults sit for more than eight hours a day, four in ten are physically inactive, and one in ten report both, according to *JAMA Network*.[9] Further research found that sitting for prolonged periods of time has been linked to an increased risk of obesity, diabetes, heart disease, dementia, and several types of cancers.[10] If you're sedentary, you also have a greater risk of an early death.[11]

But even if you exercise daily, you may not reverse the harmful health effects caused by sitting long hours every day.

Obesity expert James Levine, MD, PhD, delivered a scathing indictment about staying on your rear end for so long.

"We are sitting ourselves to death," he insists. "Sitting is more dangerous than smoking, kills more people than HIV, and is more treacherous than parachuting," adds Dr. Levine, former director of the Mayo Clinic Obesity Solutions Institute and author of *Get Up! Why Your Chair Is Killing You and What You Can Do About It*.[12]

Now let's look at some scientific conclusions:

- **If you move more, you can keep weight off over the long term.** Researchers followed nearly 200 inactive obese men and women aged sixty-five to eighty-five for six months. As the study in *Obesity* revealed, one third of the subjects did structured exercise such as treadmill workouts. The second third did what researchers called the SitLess intervention, which encourages people to stay active throughout the day by doing enjoyable activities such as walking the dog or gardening. The final group followed a weight loss program, did structured exercise, and made sure to SitLess. All three groups lost a similar amount of weight in the first six months (a little more than eighteen pounds), but those who *moved throughout the day* kept off more weight at eighteen months. "What people need to realize is that "accumulating movement across the day has benefits—and sometimes greater benefits—than a focus on only structured exercise," explains Jason Fanning, PhD, assistant professor in the Department of Health and Exercise Science at Wake Forest University in Winston-Salem, NC.[13]

- **Successful weight maintainers sat less than obese individuals.** For a study in *Obesity* that was funded by WW (formerly, Weight Watchers), researchers studying habits of more than 4,300 "weight loss maintainers" found that those who kept off the weight spent an average of three hours *less* per day sitting than "weight stable" obese people. [14]

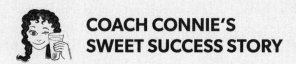

COACH CONNIE'S SWEET SUCCESS STORY

How I Sat Less, Stood More, and Did Pilates to Beat Back Pain

Are you among the 65 million Americans with a recent episode of back pain or 16 million adults with chronic or severe back pain?[15] If so, this is for you.

Until a few years ago, I was a habitual sitter. That's an occupational hazard of being a writer and author on frequent deadlines. Over time, my oversitting triggered chronic, debilitating lower back pain until it was agonizing to sit. Determined to find relief, I:

- **Got a standing desk.** Ideally, I sit for twenty minutes at a time. Then a timer reminds me to get up, raise the level of my desk, stand, stretch, lift my arms, balance on one leg at a time, sway, swivel my hips, or dance. (Admittedly, I'm still perfecting this habit.)

- **Do Pilates.** Thanks to two or more hour-long Pilates workouts a week, I've toned my core, improved my posture, and eliminated back pain.

- **Take short walks.** Not only is this great for my back, but moving improves my mindset, creativity, and peace of mind.

Join me whether or not you have back pain. Get up and start moving!

It's not about perfect. It's about effort. And when you bring that effort every single day, that's where transformation happens.[16]

—**Jillian Michaels**, fitness expert, TV personality, and author of the *New York Times* bestseller *Winning by Losing: Drop the Weight, Change Your Life*

MORE PROOF:
The Science about Exercise's Benefits

Any type of exercise is good for you. Consider:

- **Walking lowers the risk of obesity.** More than 6,000 overweight people who wore activity trackers for four years lowered their risk of obesity by 64 percent by increasing their step count from 6,000 to 11,000 per day, according to the National Institute of Health's All of Us Health Program.[17] Taking more steps also was related to decreased risk for type 2 diabetes, hypertension, depression, and sleep apnea.

- **Yoga can help you shed weight.** Although yoga doesn't burn many calories, it can help slim you down, according to a study in *Evidence-Based Complementary and Alternative Medicine*. Researchers found that yoga offers "diverse behavioral, physical, and psychosocial effects that may make it a useful tool for weight loss."[18]

- **Pilates trims stomach fat and improves moods.** A study published in *Physiology and Behavior* found that a one-hour-long Pilates session improved moods in sedentary women.[19] I can vouch for that. After doing Pilates, I always feel great!

- **Resistance training brings benefits.** Research published in the *British Journal of Sports Medicine* found that lifting weights can improve strength, shrink fat, and help build lean muscle tissue. Scientists also found a 34 percent reduction in falls among those who regularly did resistance training and balance exercises.[20]

> *If you don't make time for exercise,*
> *you'll probably have to make time for illness.*[21]

—**Robin Sharma**, leadership expert and bestselling author
of *The 5 AM Club* and *The Everyday Hero Manifesto*

FEASTS (Fast, Easy, Awesome, Simple, Tested Strategies) to Help You Move More and Sit Less

When I say exercise, I'm not talking about running five miles before dawn. Your goal is to exercise at least one half hour a day. Indeed, the recommended physical activity level is 50 to 300 minutes of moderate-intensity exercise a week, including brisk walking, dancing, doubles tennis, or water aerobics each week, plus muscle-strength or resistance training at least two days a week.[22]

If you're new to working out, here are tips to get going:

- **Start slowly.** Begin with short walks indoors, in place or on a treadmill. Take outdoor walks alone or with friends. For motivation, find a walking group. Keep your workouts short and gradually build intensity and frequency. Repeat *walkirmations* (affirmations while you walk inside or stride outside).

- **Create a balanced routine.** Do you like yoga, bicycling, tennis, pickleball, or swimming? When you match your personality to your workout, you'll be more likely to stick with it, according to a study in *Science Daily*.[23] Schedule in advance what activities you'll do on what days.

- **Drink ample water.** Before, during, and after your workout, make sure to drink one to two glasses of water.

- **Exercise to honor life.** Take the lead of athletic performance coach Brian Nguyen, who put it well: "I want to keep this vehicle clean, tuned up, and running on great fuel. That way, I can keep enjoying the open road with my loved ones!"[24]

- **Move more every day.** Stretch your arms high or to the side; balance on one leg, then the other; do squats; lift weights, hold five-second planks, or walk in place. Stretch, swirl, or spin during restroom breaks. Conduct walking meetings or get up as often as possible during live or online meetings. Always take the stairs. Invest in a standing desk, if you can, or ask your employer to provide one. Then step in place while you work.

- **Take organized classes.** Join a fitness club, take classes at a recreation center in your area, or find online classes.

The simple act of moving your body will do more for your brain than any riddle, math equation, mystery book, or even thinking itself. Exercise has numerous pro-health effects on the body—especially on the brain. It's a powerful player in the world of epigenetics.[25]

—**David Perlmutter, MD**, brain expert, neurologist, and author of such *New York Times* bestsellers as *Grain Brain* and *Drop Acid*

It's Dance Party Time!

You've now completed the first week of your Bounce Back Boldly Plan. This means it's time to celebrate. To wrap up our first seven days together, we're going to have the first of several dance parties. We're going to bop, rock, and romp.

If you love moving to music as much as I do, you know it lifts you up, invigorates you, and puts you in a triumphant mood.

Research shows that dance provides a "pleasure double play." Indeed, while you're having fun, the music will be stimulating your brain's reward centers, and boogieing will be activating your sensory and motor circuits.[26]

> *People who are regularly active have a stronger sense of purpose, and they experience more gratitude, love, and hope. They feel more connected to their communities, and are less likely to suffer from loneliness or become depressed. These benefits are seen throughout the lifespan.[27]*

—Kelly McGonigal, PhD, health psychologist and author of *The Joy of Movement: How Exercise Helps Us Find Happiness, Hope, Connection, and Courage*

For the first Dance Party of your Bounce Back Boldly Plan, I selected five tunes to gear you up for empowerment, resilience, and success.

Just pretend that we're rejoicing together while you turn on these tunes and crank up the volume. Now let's get prancing, stepping, and strutting to these uplifting songs.

- "Confident" with Demi Lovato[28]
- "Million Reasons" by Lady Gaga[29]
- "Wonderful Life" with Zendaya[30]
- "Dancing With Myself" by Billy Idol[31]
- "Rise Up" by Andra Day[32]

Pat yourself on the back that you completed Week I. Now take a well-deserved break. Weather permitting, enjoy the great outdoors either alone or with your family and/or friends.

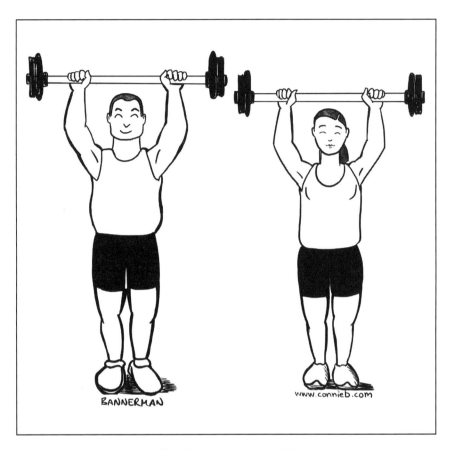

"It feels so great to work out!"

Beyond-the-Book Support:
Popular Online Workouts

For ideas on where to find online workout classes, visit my blog at www.connieb.com/Popular-Online-Workouts.

Chapter 20

Week Two

THE BOUNCE BACK
BOLDLY PLAN

*[T]he more aware you become of your spiritual being,
the more you want to respect your physical being.*

It's a spiritual diet: You love yourself too much to eat crap![1]

—**Gabrielle Bernstein**, *New York Times* bestselling author
of *Super Attractor* and *The Universe Has Your Back*

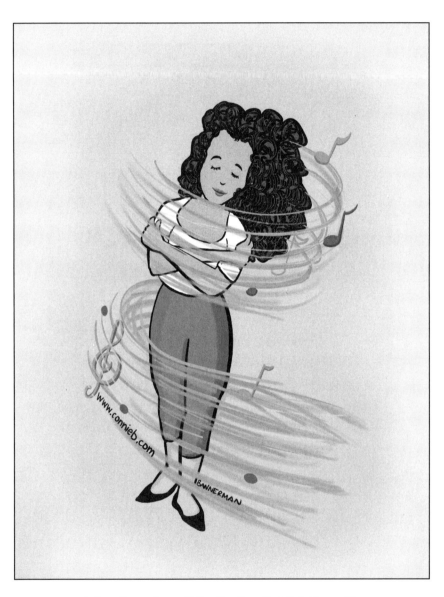

Self-soothe anytime with the *Hug-Hum-Rock Relief Process™*.

DAY 8

DO THE HUG-HUM-ROCK RELIEF PROCESS™

A hug is always the right size.[1]

—**Winnie the Pooh,** the popular fictional
teddy bear created by author A. A. Milne

Hugging.
It's one of the fastest, no-cost, powerful ways to jumpstart your journey to Bounce Back Boldly.

I'm pleased to introduce you to an easy technique which helps you self-soothe, get a healthy "high," and have fun at the same time.

Meet my Hug-Hum-Rock Relief Process, which invites you to embrace you, yourself, and you. Yes, you read that right!

With this tactic, you'll boost feelings of well-being, security, and comfort by releasing *oxytocin*, the feel-good or cuddle hormone and neurotransmitter that plays a big role in trust, social bonding, and relationship-building.[2] It's even been called the "love drug."[3]

What makes the Hug-Hum-Rock Relief Process so easy-peasy is that you can do it by and on yourself *at any time* to get those warm, fuzzy, reassuring feelings. Plus, of course, you can invite your loved ones to join you in a fun-filled Hug-Hum-Rock Relief party.

Human touch is a component of health and stress reduction that is usually underappreciated. Science has shown that touch, massage, hugging, and physical acknowledgment, in general, helps us release the feel-good hormones that keep us more prone to relaxation and stronger in the face of stress.[4]

—**Mark Hyman**, M.D., internationally recognized advocate
of Functional Medicine and *New York Times* bestselling author of
numerous books, including *Young Forever*

COACH CONNIE'S SWEET SUCCESS STORY

How I Created the Hug-Hum-Rock Relief Process

By now you know that I pigged out on lots of cruddy carbs for months after I lost my mom. One day, after months of struggling, floundering, and bingeing, I angrily resolved to escape that rut.

This time, after I drove to a nearby movie theater (I still needed to escape), my intuition told me to stay put. After parking my car, I put a favorite CD into the stereo. While the melody played, I wrapped my arms around myself and began to hug, hum, and rock to the music. After the first tune ended, I repeated the process to another song.

Five minutes later, I felt soothed, calmed, and confident enough to resist my biggest temptation—crunchy, greasy, salty movie popcorn. For the first time in months, I waltzed right by the concession stand—and easily ignored the carbage. Really!

After that first triumph, I was excited. Over and over, I began to do more hugging, humming, and rocking. *Every single time, I felt relieved, calmed, and encouraged!*

Next, I experimented at home. I caressed myself often. Then I was self-affectionate in private *before* I entered any potentially tempting or trying situations.

The more I practiced, the more I added things like stroking, squeezing, and massaging my arms, legs, butt, and belly.

Astoundingly, I've had a 100 percent success rate every time. In short, whenever I lovingly embraced myself, hummed (or sang along) to a tune, and rocked myself, my cravings vanished.

As a journalist, I was brimming with curiosity. How had I so quickly shifted from *helplessly* pigging out on carb crap to *effortlessly* ignoring the stuff?

After combing through medical studies, I unlocked the secret to this technique. The reason it worked was quite simple. All I did to ignore once-tempting carbage was combine several powerful, scientifically validated techniques—hugging, humming or singing, rocking, self-massaging, and/or self-stroking. When I did three to five of these tactics at once, I was ramping up the potency big-time by releasing a plethora of those "feel good" hormones oxytocin, dopamine, and serotonin.[5]

That's how my Hug-Hum-Rock Relief Process was born more than a decade ago at this writing. To this day, I playfully do this technique whenever I want to calm down, encourage myself, feel comforted, boost my mood, or make myself smile.

THE PROOF: The Fascinating Science That Backs the Hug-Hum-Rock-Relief Process

First, you need to know that music serves as the backbone for this technique. Let's explore some of its many benefits:

Music, Humming, and Singing

- **Music matched medications in reducing anxiety.** Music was found to be *as effective as prescription drugs* in lessening anxiety before surgery, according to a study in the journal *Regional Anesthesia & Pain Medicine*. Scientists gave one group of patients up to two milligrams of the sedative midazolam intravenously before the operation.[6] The other participants listened to Marconi Union's "Weightless," which you've been enjoying as well. Anxiety scores recorded before and after the medical procedure indicate that the sedated people and the music listeners were *equally soothed*.

- **Singing boosts immunity and makes people happier.** Crooning can cause beneficial changes in neurotransmitters and hormones, according to a review in the *Journal of Voice*. The benefits of singing included boosting oxytocin along with immunoglobulin A, which plays a crucial role in immunity, and releasing endorphins.[7] (Remember, endorphins increase feelings of happiness.)

- **Humming for just five minutes lowers your stress levels.** Researchers found that doing a slow-paced breathing exercise called *Bhramari Pranayama* (The Humming Bee Breath or Bumblebee Breath) for only five minutes lowered heart rate and blood pressure. All the subjects did was hum "O-U-Mmmma" while they exhaled with a "humming nasal sound mimicking the sound of a humming wasp," researchers explained in the *Nepal Medical College Journal*.[8]

- **Humming improves your health.** Humming for five to ten minutes at a time not only lowered stress, but it reduced heart rate, blood pressure, and pulse rate, according to a study in the *Journal of Traditional and Complementary Medicine*. Humming also improved cognition, helped with tinnitus symptoms, and even lessened anxiety, depression, and irritability.[9]

If you notice that you're feeling tense, upset or self-critical, try giving yourself a warm hug, or tenderly stroking your arm or face, or gently rocking your body.[10]

—**Kristin Neff, PhD**, researcher, University of Texas at Austin associate professor, and author of *Self-Compassion: The Proven Power of Being Kind to Yourself*

Hugging, Self-Massaging, and Stroking

Now we come to the second part of the Hug-Hum-Rock Relief Process. Research points to the therapeutic effects of touching others or yourself. For instance:

- **Self-soothing touch gestures such as putting your hand on your heart offers protective effects on stress.** Research in *Comprehensive Psychoneuroendocrinology* suggested that receiving hugs and "self-soothing touch gestures reduce cortisol responses to psychosocial stress." The findings also "suggest that self-soothing touch and receiving hugs are simple and yet potentially powerful means for buffering individuals' resilience against stress."[11]
- **Hugging triggers oxytocin among women.** A study of premenopausal women published in *Biological Psychology* found that the subjects' oxytocin levels rose after frequent hugs from their partners. Those changes were associated with lower blood pressure and heart rate.[12]
- **Getting hugs helps people shake off challenges.** Scientists who studied more than 400 healthy adults found that both men and women who were hugged didn't remain as upset by interpersonal conflicts as those who weren't clasped, according to research published in *PLOS One*. In short, hugging acted like a buffer against stress.[13]

Teddy Bears Aren't Just for Kids

The next time you yearn for instant peace, comfort, and security, try cuddling a teddy bear. Seriously! You may think, "That's for kids!" But did you know that more than half of American adults still have a favorite teddy bear?[14]

You guessed it. Hugging your teddy bear lifts your spirits by releasing those feel-good hormones oxytocin and serotonin.[15]

- **Self-massage helps people soothe stress and quit smoking.** A study published in the *Journal of Child and Adolescent Substance Abuse* studied smokers who wanted to quit. Half the participants did self-massage and received coaching in believing in themselves. The remaining subjects got guidance on giving up smoking. The stress and daily smoking levels of self-massagers improved immediately and remained that way four weeks later. The control group showed no improvements.[16]

The Calming Pet Effect

Science reveals that ten minutes of hugging, stroking, or touching your pet can lower the stress hormone cortisol and increase levels of oxytocin.[17] A study of nearly 250 college students published in *AERA Open* by the American Educational Research Association found that those who petted and played with cats or dogs during a ten-minute, college-based animal visitation program with shelter animals had a sizeable drop in cortisol levels. Not so with those who watched a slideshow of the animals or waited for their turn to touch the animals. Goofing off with pets is so successful in helping students manage stress due to academic demands that Animal Visitation Programs are in place at nearly 1,000 US college campuses.[18]

Rocking

For the last part of the Hug-Hum-Rock Relief Process, we'll look at two types of rocking:

- **Rocking to music makes people happier.** A study in the *Psychology of Music* found that participants who went out dancing or attended music events were the happiest. "People who intentionally interact with music [are] using an outlet to express their emotions," pointed out study coauthor Melissa Weinberg, PhD.[19]
- **You can rock away your pain.** Rocking in chairs reduced depression and anxiety in nursing home patients with dementia, according to research published in the *American Journal of Alzheimer's Disease*. In a six-week test, patients rocked an average of 101 minutes a day. Another benefit: The more participants rocked, the more they were able to cut back on pain medication.[20]
- **Rocking can calm you down.** Women suffering from fibromyalgia experienced increased feelings of peace and relief and got help managing their pain by rocking in chairs ten minutes a day, three times a week, for sixteen weeks, according to a study in *Dignified and Purposeful Living for Older Adults*.[21]

FEASTS (Fast, Easy, Awesome, Simple, Tested Strategies) to do the Hug-Hum-Rock Relief Process

Drum roll, please. I'm delighted to tell you how to practice my enjoyable Hug-Hum-Rock Relief Process:

- **First, find tunes you like.** Decide what kind of music you need in that moment. Do you want to feel soothed, reassured, or energized? Choose melodies that match the mood you seek. For instance, if you lost a loved one, check out the comforting tunes "Mama" from Il Divo[22], "Goodbye's the Saddest Word" from Celine Dion[23], or "To Where You Are" with Josh Groban.[24]
- **Hug, hum, rock, and self-massage yourself.** Stand, sit, or lie down in a private area and listen to one or more favorite tunes. Now do what feels best. Wrap your arms around your neck, back, or shoulders. Massage, stroke, or caress your head, hands, or arms. Sway, swirl, and swivel to the music. Cuddle yourself for as long as you like.

- **Rock on.** If you're feeling energetic, start dancing at the same time. Or move in other ways that feel fun.
- **Pick and play tunes** *before* **temptation strikes.** Plan ahead. Whenever you go to a grocery store, movie theater, or family gathering where junk foods are available, decide *in advance* that you'll make smart choices. Before you leave home, listen to one or more of your favorite tunes on your preferred device while you do the Hug-Hum-Rock Relief Process.
- **Find a Personal Power Anthem.** You know how sports teams use head-bopping, foot-stomping, hand-clapping songs to hype up their fans before a big game? Choose your very own *Personal Power Anthem* to boost your spirits while you do the Hug-Hum-Rock-Relief Process. Try listening, for instance, to "Girl on Fire" by Alicia Keys[25], "Just Dance" by Lady Gaga[26], or "Roar" by Katy Perry.[27]

Now have fun practicing and personalizing this easy, powerful, science-based Hug-Hum-Rock Relief Process and get lifted to a calmer, cozier, happier place.

Beyond-the-Book Support:
Get My Bounce Back Boldly Boogie Playlist

To help you get the most out of the Hug-Hum-Rock Relief Process, I've compiled a Bounce Back Boldly Boogie Playlist on Spotify. It features more than 100 tunes from a variety of genres, including choral, classical, country, electronic, jazz, operatic, pop, and rock. Find out how to access my Spotify playlist at www.BounceBackDiet.com/Book-Bonuses.

DAY 9

ENJOY WATER'S WONDERS

*Drinking water is like taking a shower
on the inside of your body.[1]*

—Unknown

For decades people have been trying to find a way to drink away pounds using a variety of meal-replacement shakes.

But what if I told you that there's a simple elixir that can help you drop off the weight? A beverage that will make you feel fuller, burn fat and calories without any effort, and crank up your metabolism? What if I told you that you were already drinking this wonder drink—but probably not enough?

Of course, this miracle beverage is water.

Water's Vital Role in Our Health

Why is drinking water so important? Well, our bodies are made up of about 60 percent water, so you want to keep up levels of H_2O to make your body run better.[2]

Water increases our energy, helps improve cognitive function, facilitates digestion, helps maintain blood pressure, keeps muscles healthy, assists in flushing waste through urination, balances our body's chemicals, lubricates and cushions joints, regulates body temperature, boosts skin health, reduces depression, makes minerals and nutrients accessible, improves our immune system, and may prevent memory decline.[3]

On the other hand, not getting enough water leads to dehydration and a host of symptoms, including headaches, mental confusion, fatigue, dizziness, lightheadedness, dry mouth, muscle cramps, swollen feet, the chills, constipation, and sugar cravings.[4] Chronic dehydration may even result in altered kidney, heart, or digestive function.[5] And without water, we human beings would survive for only about three days.[6]

THE PROOF:
The Fascinating Science about Water's Role in Shedding Weight

Let's look at research that shows how water can help you shed and keep off weight:

- **People who don't drink enough water weigh more.** A study published in *The Annals of Family Medicine* looked at more than 9,000 people aged eighteen to sixty-four and found that adults who didn't hydrate adequately were more likely to be obese compared to those who drank enough.[7]

- **Preloading with water before a meal helps pounds slide off.** A study in *Obesity* looked at nearly 200 overweight premenopausal women and found that when the female subjects increased daily water consumption to thirty-four or more ounces (about 4¼ eight-ounce glasses) and made no other changes to their diet or lifestyles, they lost more than four pounds a year on average.[8]

- **Drinking water instead of diet soda helps with weight loss.** In a study published in the *International Journal of Obesity*, participants who swapped water for diet beverages lost more weight, had lower BMIs, and maintained lower fasting insulin levels after six months compared to those who drank diet beverages.[9]

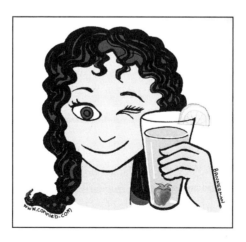

Discover the wonders of water.

Eco-Friendly Pointer: Skip Plastic Bottles

While you want to drink filtered water for your health, don't chug it out of plastic bottles. Americans buy about 50 billion plastic water bottles every year, and the average person disposes of some thirteen plastic bottles per month.[10] But if you use a reusable bottle instead, you'll save some 156 plastic bottles a year.[11]

Unfortunately, only about 9 percent of plastic is recycled, so most bottles end up in landfills.[12] Plastic breaks down into microscopic particles or microplastics according to *Environmental Science and Pollution Research*. These can contaminate soil and waterways and be ingested by fish, seabirds, aquatic creatures, and later, us humans.[13]

Plastic water bottles also may contain bisphenol-A, or BPA, which research suggests may seep into beverages or foods. The Mayo Clinic points to "a possible link between BPA and increased blood pressure, type 2 diabetes, and cardiovascular disease."[14]

The solution? Invest in one or more reusable bottles made of stainless steel or glass. Carry one with you wherever you go, refill it often, and drink to your health and that of the planet.

FEASTS (Fast, Easy, Awesome, Simple, Tested Strategies) to Drink Water for Weight Loss and Better Health

It's time to drink up.

- **Find out how much water you need every day.** The general rule of thumb is to drink at least half your body weight in ounces. Once you calculate how much H_2O you need, divide that figure by eight to get the number of eight-ounce glasses to drink throughout the day. (If, for instance, you weigh 160 pounds, you want to drink eighty ounces or ten eight-ounce glasses of water a day.)[15]

- **Sip often.** At the start of the day, pour filtered water into one or more containers. Keep refilling your carafe(s) until you meet your requirement.
- **Drink one to two glasses of water a half hour before every meal.**[16]
- **Always bring water with you.** Whenever you head out the door, bring an eco-friendly water bottle with you.
- **Find out if you're hydrated.** First, you can check the color of your urine. If your pee is a pale straw yellow color, you're hydrated.[17] Another way to know if you're hydrated is to pinch the skin on your arm between two fingers. When you let go, if your skin springs back to its normal appearance within a second or two, you have skin turgor or skin elasticity. That means you've had enough water.[18]
- **Add some flavor.** To spruce up the taste of water, add slices of ginger, orange, lemon, lime, berries, cucumber, or herbal tea bags.

Are you in the mood yet? For water, of course. Speaking of which, now is a good time to get a reusable, eco-friendly, metal or glass bottle. For ideas, see the list of Eco-Friendly Water Bottles in the Recommended Resources section on page 324 so you always have ample water with you when you're on the go.[19]

DAY 10

BOOST YOUR BODY IMAGE WITH DAILY GRATITUDE

Gratitude begins in our hearts and then dovetails into behavior. It almost always makes you willing to be of service, which is where the joy resides When you are aware of all that has been given to you in your lifetime and the past few days, it is hard not to be humbled, and pleased to give back.[1]

—**Anne Lamott,** *New York Times* bestselling author of
Somehow, Bird by Bird, and *Dusk, Night, Dawn*

We're often bombarded by photos of women and men with unrealistically slim, toned bodies, as well as impossibly flawless skin, silky hair, and not an itty-bitty wrinkle in sight. Since most pictures have been airbrushed, photoshopped, or retouched, it can be discouraging to see those perfect images on Instagram, Facebook, and the Web, or in magazines.[2]

Take heart. Gratitude can save the day. Indeed, thankfulness—which has been linked to lower rates of depression and anxiety, improved health, better sleep, and more fulfilling relationships—also can help you feel better about your body.[3]

Gratitude places you in the energy field of plentitude. Perceiving life in a consciousness of gratitude is literally stepping into another dimension of living. Suddenly the seeming ordinariness of your days takes on a divine sparkle.[4]

—**Michael Beckwith,** minister, founder and spiritual director
of Agape International Spiritual Center

THE PROOF: The Fascinating Science about How Gratitude Improves Body Satisfaction

Studies have shown that the more we appreciate our body, the more likely we are to treat it well by listening to its needs and nourishing it with better foods. Consider:

- **Gratitude bolsters body appreciation.** Women with higher levels of gratitude were *less concerned* about other people's opinions of their appearance, which, in turn, made them *appreciate themselves* *more and eat healthier*, according to research published in the journal *Body Image*. For the study, nearly 300 women completed questionnaires about gratitude, image, social comparison, and intuitive eating, which is when you eat due to hunger. The results suggest that by "amplifying the good in their own lives, gratitude helps to direct women's sense of self-worth toward other positive aspects of their lives," observed lead researcher Kristin J. Homan, PhD, a psychology professor at Grove City College in Pennsylvania. "This awareness of what is good about one's body will lead the individual to value the body more, and to treat it in a way that will enhance it."[5]

- **Thankfulness makes you appreciate your body more.** Another study in *Body Image* found that reframing the way we think about our bodies can improve our opinions about them. For the research, half of the female participants were told to consider and write about three aspects of their body for which they felt grateful such as their health, physical characteristics, or how their body functions. Those instructed to feel grateful were *more accepting* of their bodies regardless of their weight.[6]

> *Spend two minutes a day scanning the world for three new things you're grateful for. And do that for 21 days. The reason why that's powerful is you're training your brain to scan the world in a new pattern. You're scanning for positives, instead of scanning for threats. It's the fastest way of teaching optimism.*[7]
>
> —**Shawn Achor**, *New York Times* bestselling author of *The Happiness Advantage* and founder of GoodThink

MORE PROOF: Gratitude Also Helps Your Health

- **Being thankful helps you stay fit.** People who practiced gratitude for ten weeks were more likely to exercise nearly one-and-a-half more hours per week than a control group, according to a study in the *Journal of Personality and Social Psychology*.[8]
- **Gratitude improves physical health.** Researchers found a link between people who expressed gratitude and good physical health. After studying nearly 1,000 adults aged nineteen to eighty-four, scientists noticed that giving thanks led people to appreciate and

take better care of their bodies, according to a study in the journal *Personality and Individual Differences.*[9]

- **Giving thanks enhances sleep.** Writing in a gratitude journal for fifteen minutes every evening can reduce worry at bedtime and promote longer and better sleep, according to a study in *Applied Psychology Health and Well-Being.*[10]

> *Gratitude is the key to happiness. When gratitude is practiced regularly and from the heart, it leads to a richer, fuller and more complete life.*[11]
>
> —**Vishen Lakhiani**, founder/CEO of www.Mindvalley.com and *New York Times* bestselling author of *The Buddha and the Badass* and *The Code of the Extraordinary Mind*

FEASTS (Fast, Easy, Awesome, Simple, Tested Strategies) to Boost Your Body Image with Gratitude

Begin now to give thanks daily for your awesome body. Here are some ways to start:

- **Speak kindly to your body.** Think and say positive things about your body. If you like, share these statements with a close friend or loved one.
- **Pause and pivot.** If you ever forget the wonders of your body, stop and then give thanks for your remarkable vessel.
- **Create Body Appreciation Affirmations.** Ramp up acceptance for your amazing body by joyfully giving thanks. Here are three ideas:

  I am feeling grateful for my healthy body.
  I appreciate my amazing body.
  I am loving my awesome body.

- **Put your thanks in writing.** Start or end your day writing down three to five things for which you're thankful. Single out parts of your body that you like most and least. Focus on the amazing things your body lets you do, not what it looks like. Write about other things you appreciate, too.

- **Cook with gratitude.** When you prepare meals, be thankful for the sunshine, the rain, and the farmers who planted and picked the real foods at your meal.
- **Say grace.** To help you shift your attention to the blessings in your life, give thanks for your meal(s) before you eat. You'll be joining 48 percent of all Americans who say grace several times a week.[12]

> *To say grace before meals is, among other things, to remember that it was God, not my credit card, that provided my meal.*[13]
>
> **—Lauren F. Winner**, historian, Episcopal priest, writer, and associate professor of Christian Spirituality at Duke Divinity School

- **Boost your willpower with gratitude.** If you're ever tempted by junk foods, immediately think or write about three or more things for which you're thankful.
- **Take Gratitude Walks.** While you stroll outdoors, be grateful for the many beautiful sights around you. And appreciate your body, which allows you to move around.

You now have a beautiful gratitude habit. To close, let's thank our bodies for their dedicated service to us.

Gratitude for Our Amazing Bodies

Thank you, dear body, for always being there for me.
I am grateful that you allow me to breathe, move, love,
and live. Amen.

DAY 11

WRITE YOUR WAY TO WELLNESS

We should write because . . . writing is a powerful form of prayer and meditation, connecting us both to our own insights and to a higher and deeper level of inner guidance. . . . We should write because writing brings clarity and passion to the act of living. . . . We should write because writing is good for the soul.[1]

—**Julia Cameron,** author of the bestselling guide,
The Artist's Way: A Spiritual Path to Higher Creativity

In the bestselling novel *Bridget Jones's Diary*, the endearing, self-mocking, thirty-two-year-old fictional character kept a diary to manage her life. In her daily entries, Bridget shared poignant, humorous, provocative observations about men, food, exercise, sex, and her wildly fluctuating weight.[2]

". . . I am a child of *Cosmopolitan* culture, have been traumatized by super-models and too many quizzes and know that neither my personality nor my body is up to it if left to its own devices. I can't take the pressure," the make-believe Bridget wrote.

·Clearly, women worldwide have identified with Bridget's concerns. The wildly successful novel by Helen Fielding has sold more than fifteen million copies in forty countries and spawned three romantic comedies with Renée Zellweger, Colin Firth, and Hugh Grant.[3]

Write what disturbs you, what you fear, what you have not been willing to speak about. Be willing to be split open.[4]

—**Natalie Goldberg**, advocate of writing as a Zen practice and author of the bestseller, *Writing Down the Bones: Freeing the Writer Within*

You, Too, Can Write Away Your Worries

What does the make-believe Bridget Jones have to do with you? Today you'll begin to find out how writing can help you Bounce Back Boldly.

Putting your ideas, thoughts, and feelings on paper is a powerful way to process them and become your best, boldest, brightest self. Writing also can help you heal. It's easy, fast, and free—other than the price of paper or a journal. And you don't even need to be a good writer.

For starters, penning words on the page is cathartic. Writing also helps you analyze roadblocks, identify your triggers, and puts things into perspective.

[Journaling has] really helped me get an idea of what my behaviors are, what my patterns are, how I can make change for myself for good. It made me be honest with myself. Now it's part of my daily habits, like brushing my teeth.[5]

—**Charmaine Jackson**, who credits writing down what she ate with helping her go from 260 pounds to 130 pounds

THE PROOF: The Fascinating Science about Keeping a Journal or a Food Diary

Let the following research convince you to pick up pen or pencil pronto:

- **You get beneficial changes in your brain by writing about painful incidents.** Psychologist Matthew Lieberman, PhD and his team from the University of California at Los Angles discussed positive effects from writing about past negative experiences for their study in *Social Cognitive and Affective Neuroscience*. Brain scans taken three months after people started journaling showed that the writers had greater activity in specific areas of the brain, especially the prefrontal cortex. This means that putting thoughts and feelings into words may lead to better physical health and life satisfaction, as well as less depression and anxiety.[6]
- **If you consistently keep a food diary, you may lose more weight.** Now let's turn to another kind of writing. A study published in the *American Journal of Preventive Medicine* found that those people who kept a food diary six days a week lost about *twice as much weight* as those who only kept track of what they ate just one day or less each week.[7]

Journaling is the perfect way to shift your emotions immediately and process your feelings without judgment, so you don't get stuck in unpleasant experiences.[8]

—**Kristen Butler,** author of the *3 Minute Positivity Journal* and the Power of Positivity founder/CEO, who once weighed 331 pounds and "lost half" of herself

FEASTS (Fast, Easy, Awesome, Simple, Tested Strategies) to Write Your Way to Wellness

It's time to test out the power of the pen:

- **Write "Morning Pages."** Creativity teacher Julia Cameron, author of *The Artist's Way*, recommends stream-of-consciousness writing by longhand first thing in the morning until you fill three 8½" × 11" pages. "Nothing is too petty, too silly, too stupid or too weird to be included," she explains. "Once we get those muddy, maddening, confusing thoughts [nebulous worries, jitters, and pre-occupations] on the page, we face our day with clearer eyes."[9]

- **Try expressive writing for twenty minutes.** If you've had a tough time, put down your thoughts and feelings on paper about what upset, embarrassed, or worried you. Even three days of jotting things down will help. Then reflect. What did you learn? What can you do about it? When you write about your grief, trauma, or other emotions, you can "stand back and reevaluate issues in your life," points out Dr. James W. Pennebaker, advocate of expressive writing or therapeutic journaling and author of *Opening Up by Writing It Down*.[10]

- **Draw instead of write.** If you prefer, sketch about what's on your mind. Have fun with it. Angry at unhealthy but tempting, cunning carbs and other junk foods? Turn them into odious characters.

- **Write away your cravings.** Can't get that bagel, sweet roll, or pizza out of your mind? Set down your thoughts about why those junk foods are beckoning. Then delve deeper. What's *really* bugging you?

- **Upset? Do Rant Writing.** If you're especially rankled, try what I call *Rant Writing*. This is a way to quickly scribble by hand or even pound away on the computer while you constructively rage, rant, and seethe. Of course, no one needs to know about your literary temper tantrum!

- **Keep a Food-and-Mood Diary.** Jot down what, how much, and where you ate and how you felt. Approach your food diary "with an attitude of nonjudgment," suggests Susan Albers, PsyD, a psychologist at the Cleveland Clinic and author of *Hanger Management*. "Commit to leaving your inner critic out of it. Look at it like conducting an experiment and you are gathering helpful data."[11]

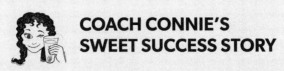

COACH CONNIE'S SWEET SUCCESS STORY

Writing Helped Me Heal and Peel Off Pounds

Admittedly, I'm biased, because I'm a professional writer and author, but I've found tremendous relief, eye-opening insights, and much-needed peace of mind just by putting my thoughts, feelings, and worries on paper.

Take Chapter 1 in this book, where I recounted my tale of Heartbreak Bingeing after the grueling time with my dying mother. Over the years, I wrote and edited my story dozens, if not hundreds, of times. At first, I cried a lot while writing. My unprocessed emotions kept bubbling to the surface.

Finally, one day, I calmly edited it. No tears. That's when I knew I'd finally healed. Journaling or writing is that powerful.

It's your turn. Take a pen or pencil in hand and start writing or drawing in your journal to heal your heart, scribble away your woes, and connect with your smart self.

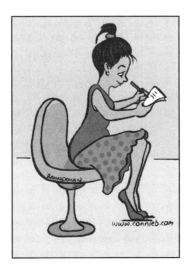

It's time to write your way to wellness.

DAY 12

EAT DINNER EARLIER AND SKIP LATE-NIGHT GRAZING

I rarely have treats around that might tempt me late at night, which is when I usually crave something really fattening. What am I going to do? Drive out at 11 at night just to satisfy a craving? No, that's crazy.[1]

—**Jennifer Love Hewitt,** actress, singer/songwriter, and producer

Most of us know all about the unhealthy habit of *Late-Night Grazing*. This is when you chomp on chips, crackers, or other nutrient-lacking foods less than three hours before bedtime.

If you do nighttime snacking, you're in good company. Sixty-seven percent of Americans snack in the evening or late at night, according to a survey from the International Food Information Council.[2]

Late-Night Grazing

You're not hungry. Doesn't matter. While you watch TV or your favorite streaming service or scroll on social media, you mindlessly snack at 10 p.m., 11 p.m., or later.

THE PROOF: The Fascinating Science about The Dangers of Late-Night Grazing

Studies show that eating later can pack on pounds:

- **You're more likely to become obese when you eat more later in the day.** In a study published in the journal *PLOS One*, researchers shared their findings that folks who ate *almost half* of their daily calories during dinner were roughly *twice as likely* to become obese.[3]

- **Eating later led to increased hunger and risk of obesity.** Having a late dinner may slow down your metabolism, make you hungrier the next day, and lead to weight gain, according to Harvard Medical School investigators at Brigham and Women's Hospital. As they observed in their study in the journal *Cell Metabolism*, eating later had "profound effects on hunger and the appetite-regulating hormones leptin and grehlin."[4]

- **Late eating may lead to health issues and shedding fewer pounds.** After looking at the eating habits of nearly 3,400 adults, researchers writing in the *American Journal of Clinical Nutrition* suggested that late eating is associated with an increase in the risk of developing cardiac and metabolic disorders, shedding less weight, and being less likely to be motivated.[5]

Human circadian rhythms in sleep and metabolism are synchronized to the daily rotation of the earth, so that when the sun goes down you are supposed to be sleeping, not eating. When sleep and eating are not aligned with the body's internal clock, it can lead to changes in appetite and metabolism, which could lead to weight gain.[6]

—Phyllis C. Zee, MD, PhD, director of the Center for Circadian and Sleep Medicine and Chief of the Division of Sleep Medicine at Northwestern University Feinberg School of Medicine

Let's turn our attention now to the benefits of consuming more food earlier in the day:

- **When you eat earlier in the day, you shed more weight and inches.** Research published in the *Journal of the American College of Nutrition* looked at two groups of women who ate identical diets. The females who took in more calories during the first half of the day lost more weight and had better metabolic activity than ladies who consumed most of their food in the evening. On average, earlier eaters lost 3.75 pounds more and trimmed 33 percent more off their waistlines.[7]

FEASTS (Fast, Easy, Awesome, Simple, Tested Strategies) to Cut Out Late-Night Eating or Grazing

- **Eat more earlier in the day.** You'll be less likely to indulge late at night and find it easier to maintain a healthier weight.[8]
- **Stop eating three hours before bedtime.** Pick a time when you'll end your last meal of the day. Then don't eat for about eleven to twelve hours between dinnertime and breakfast the next morning. If you go to bed at 10 p.m., stop eating by 7 p.m. Or, if you get shut-eye at 11 p.m., end dinner by 8 p.m.
- **Leave the kitchen.** After dinner, wash the dishes, and make your kitchen and dining room off limits.
- **Brush your teeth.** Soon after dinner, brush and floss your teeth. This helps you remember that you're done eating for the day.
- **After dinner, drink tea.** If you'd like a "treat," try a cup of herbal tea.
- **Take a walk after dinner.** If you can, go for a stroll after your evening meal. This will get your mind off food and keep your metabolism humming. If it's cold, rainy, or snowy, walk in place in your living room.

Today I invite you to begin the healthy habit of eating dinner at least three hours before bedtime. Before long, you'll prefer healthy, wholesome, early-evening meals. Soon, your diminishing waistline will thank you.

DAY 13

TAME SUBTLE ENABLERS AND FIND AN ACCOUNTABILITY BUDDY

Sometimes, no matter how much work you do on yourself and how forgiving you are and how skilled you get at letting it go, there's just no way around it: Some people are just too committed to their own dysfunction. They're painful to be around. You'd rather cover yourself with the fleas of a thousand camels than go out for a cup of coffee with them.[1]

—**Jen Sincero**, life coach and witty author of the #1 *New York Times* bestseller *You are a Badass: How to Stop Doubting Your Greatness and Start Living an Awesome Life*

Wouldn't it be nice if all your loved ones, friends, and coworkers rooted for you to shed your excess weight? Sorry to say, but usually not everyone in your life will be on board.

Instead, you may be surrounded by well-meaning Subtle Enablers, who often urge you to "have some dessert" or other junk foods. Although these people may have good intentions, their well-meaning prodding can derail your diet.

Before you identify these people, let's cut them lots of slack. Like you, they face frequent temptations in the Junk-Foods Jungle. They also may have their own dramas or traumas. They, too, may feel addicted to sweets, carbage, or fast foods.

But Subtle Enablers can doom your weight loss efforts. In fact, a landmark study in the *New England Journal of Medicine* found that a person's chance of becoming obese increases by 57 percent if a close friend is obese, 40 percent if a sibling is obese, and 37 percent if a spouse is obese.[2]

If *Peer Pressure Eating* is one reason you blew your diet, you want to identify the three types of Subtle Enablers who can dissuade, distract, or discourage you from your health goals:

- **Polite Food Pushers.** These insistent, often clueless, but hospitable folks may not realize that if you eat a few bites of dessert or a couple of French fries, you could end up going on a binge.
- **Toxic Saboteurs.** These people may have unsuccessfully tried to shed weight themselves. They may be fixated on the short term

(having certain junk foods) and not the long term (getting a healthier body).

- *Energy Vampires.* These self-involved folks can be charming, compelling, and charismatic, but they "don't recognize the needs and feelings of others," and may "feel superior" to them, according to women's health expert Christiane Northrup, MD.[3]

> *[U]ntil we can learn to stop taking the energy of others and draining our own, we're apt to do two things:*
>
> *(1) be attracted to sugar, carbs, and/or alcohol; and*
>
> *(2) keep weight on no matter what we do—even if we stop eating carbs.[4]*
>
> —**Christiane Northrup, MD**, ob-gyn and *New York Times* bestselling author of *Dodging Energy Vampires*

THE PROOF: The Fascinating Science about *Supportive Allies* and *Accountability Buddies*

Research shows that you'll be more successful at shedding pounds when you have understanding friends, encouraging family members, and sympathetic coworkers who cheer you on. I call these people *Supportive Allies.* Let's look at some promising studies that show the benefits of having such wonderful folks in your corner:

- **People who get support from a group shed more weight.** A review in *Applied Psychology Health and Well-Being* found that people in weight loss programs lost 7.7 pounds more on average in six months than those with no such support.[5]
- **Folks with weight-loss buddies are more successful at peeling off pounds.** For a study of 704 people in a fifteen-week online weight-loss program, researchers found that those people with buddies shed more weight and inches. The study in the *Journal of Health Communication* discovered that a "combination of high accepting and high challenging messages from buddies" was associated with the greatest decrease in BMI and the biggest reduction in waist size. The scientists also observed that having "a supportive buddy who was not a romantic partner was just as effective as turning to a romantic partner for assistance."[6]

- **A supportive partner facilitates weight loss.** When one member of a couple commits to losing weight, the other partner generally sheds pounds too, even if the other person isn't trying to slim down, according to a study in the journal *Obesity* that was funded by WW (formerly Weight Watchers).[7]
- **Support from online groups helps members shed weight.** Virtual support can be invaluable, according to a retrospective study in *Scientific Reports*. After analyzing data spanning two years, investigators found that nearly 78 percent of users of the Noom weight loss app were successful at slimming down.[8]

FEASTS (Fast, Easy, Awesome, Simple, Tested Strategies) to Build a Support Network While You Shed Pounds

It's time to lay the groundwork to get the support you need:

- **Identify the three types of Subtle Enablers in your life.** Write down names of people who qualify.

  Polite Food Pushers _____

  Toxic Saboteurs _____

  Energy Vampires _____

Now decide if or how to keep them at a distance if you can.

- **Identify your Supportive Allies.** List three loved ones, friends, or advocates who will encourage you to reach your weight loss goals and honor your requests to stop offering you junk foods:

  _____

  _____

  _____

Now tell them you'd like their support while you follow the Bounce Back Boldly Plan and the companion Bounce Back Diet.

- **Find an Accountability Buddy.** Join a live or online support group where you can find people with similar health-and-wellness goals. Look for walking, bicycling, or other exercise groups in your area. Find these people on Meetup or Facebook, or in weight loss groups, hospitals, and community centers in your area. Of course, you also can connect with such folks at your gym, in yoga classes, or in pickup pickleball games.
- **Text to Motivate.** Check in daily via text with your Accountability Buddy.

You'll soon find that with Supportive Allies cheering you on, it'll be much easier to stay on track.

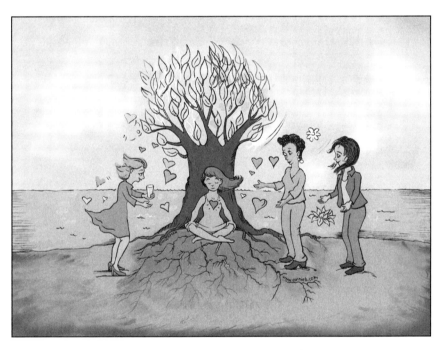

Your Supportive Allies and Accountability Buddies are vital to your success.

DAY 14

SLEEP OFF THE WEIGHT

The way to a more productive, more inspired,
more joyful life is getting enough sleep.[1]

—**Arianna Huffington,** bestselling author of *The Sleep Revolution*,
Huffington Post cofounder, and CEO of Thrive Global

How many hours of sleep do you get each night? Six? Less? In fact, more than 35 percent of Americans are sleep-deprived, getting less than seven hours of sleep a night.[2]

If you're not getting enough sleep, "you may be at an increased risk for obesity, type 2 diabetes, high blood pressure, heart disease and stroke, poor mental health, and even early death," according to the CDC.[3]

Since you're here to release unhealthy excess pounds, you want to know about research which finds that the less you slumber, the more weight you may gain.

When you don't get enough zzzs, "your metabolism will not function properly," points out clinical psychologist and sleep specialist Michael J. Breus, PhD, author of the bestselling book *The Sleep Doctor's Diet Plan: Lose Weight through Better Sleep.*

"Everything that you can do, you do better with a good night's rest."[4]

THE PROOF:
The Fascinating Science about Sleep

Let's dig into some research:

- **Less than seven hours of sleep is linked to weight gain.** A review published in *BMJ Open Sport & Exercise Medicine* found that people who got fewer than seven hours of zzzs per night were more likely to have higher body mass indexes or develop obesity than people who slept more. Sleep deprivation was linked with higher levels of *ghrelin* (the hormone that triggers hunger), inflammatory markers, and salt retention, as well as decreased levels of insulin sensitivity and *leptin* (which tells you when you're full).[5]
- **Brain scans show that sleep deprivation increases hunger for junk foods.** Scientists at the University of California at Berke-

ley scanned the brains of healthy people after a good night's sleep and then again after a night of sleep deprivation. The study, which was published in *Nature Communications*, also found that not enough shut-eye was related to an increase in brain activity relating to the *desire for high-calorie foods.*[6]

- **The less you sleep, the more you may weigh.** After surveying 1,600 adults, scientists observed that those who got six hours or less of sleep per night were, on average, one inch larger around the waist than those who slept nine hours. The study, which was published in *PLOS One*, found that people gained one pound more if they slept one less hour each night, that is, for instance, six hours instead of the recommended seven.[7]

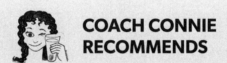

COACH CONNIE RECOMMENDS

Use Blue-Blocker Glasses at Night to Sleep Better

Electronic devices such as TVs, computers, tablets, and smart phones produce high levels of blue light, which suppresses production of the sleep-promoting hormone melatonin and may make it harder to fall asleep.[8] Excess blue light also may cause headaches, eye strain, and macular degeneration.[9]

If you'd still like to use your favorite tech gadgets at night, try one of my favorite sleep hacks—wear blue-blocker glasses. The amber-or-yellow-tinted lenses are designed to block light on the blue portion of the spectrum before it can reach your retina.

For vendor ideas, see pages 324 to 325 of the Recommended Resources section.

FEASTS (Fast, Easy, Awesome, Simple, Tested Strategies) to Sleep Better

- **Start a daily routine.** Go to bed at the same time every night and wake up at the same time every morning. Even on weekends.
- **Create a transition time before bedtime.** Spend at least a half hour getting ready for sleep. Read a book. Listen to soft music. Take a bubble bath.
- **Exercise earlier.** To sleep better, wait at least ninety minutes after you do moderate intensity exercise before you head to bed.[10]
- **Cut off coffee.** Don't drink any beverages with caffeine at least six hours before bedtime.[11]
- **Leave your cell phone out of your bedroom.** Unless you need your mobile phone by your side at all times due to, say, a family emergency, keep it in another room—ideally turned off. Arianna Huffington, author of *The Sleep Foundation: Transforming Your Life, One Night at a Time,* recommends a nightly ritual where you "gently escort" your electronic devices out of your bedroom and put your gadgets "to bed" to help you unplug.[12]
- **Make your bedroom a sacred sleep space.** Keep your room dark, because even the glow from a clock can disrupt your slumber.[13] Wear a black-out sleep mask. And set your thermostat to between 60 and 68 degrees Fahrenheit so you won't be too cold or hot.[14]
- **If sleep doesn't come, do EFT.** Tapping may help promote deep, restful sleep.
- **Consider supplements.** To help you unwind, you may want to take supplements such as GABA, L-theanine, 5-HTP, melatonin, and/or magnesium.[15] Of course, talk to your doctor first.
- **Sniff lavender.** Smelling essential oils can help you unwind before bedtime. Try lavender, ylang ylang, chamomile, bergamot, sandalwood, or marjoram oil.[16]

Wishing you sweet dreams!

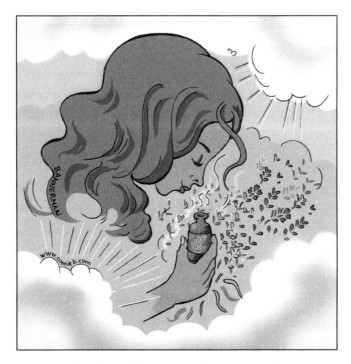

"Aaaah! I love smelling lavender before bedtime."

Hurrah! You Wrapped Up Week Two

You've now completed two weeks of the Bounce Back Boldly Plan and the companion Bounce Back Diet. You're well on your way to getting more energy, joy, and improved health.

As we conclude Week Two together, it's time to celebrate. You know what comes next. It's Dance Party Time! Put on comfortable workout clothes. Find a clear space. Now get moving to these tunes:

- "On Top Of The World" by Imagine Dragons[17]
- "Stronger" ("What Doesn't Kill You") by Kelly Clarkson[18]
- "Halo" with Beyoncé[19]
- "Dance Monkey" by Tones and I[20]
- "A Million Dreams" from the film, "The Greatest Showman," with Hugh Jackman, Michelle Williams, and Ziv Zaifman[21]

I'll be sending you encouraging thoughts while I'm off on a daily walk outdoors. See you soon, as we conclude our last week together.

Chapter 21

Week Three

THE BOUNCE BACK
BOLDLY PLAN

Perseverance is power.[1]

—Anonymous

DAY 15

BUST STRESS WITH THE CORTISOL-CALMING QUICKIE

Whenever you become anxious or stressed, outer purpose has taken over, and you lost sight of your inner purpose.[1]

—Eckhart Tolle, spiritual teacher, *New York Times* bestselling author of *The Power of Now* and *A New Earth: Awakening to Your Life's Purpose*

Stress is inevitable. No one sails through life without having a lousy day, tense disagreements with a loved one, and dozens of large or small aggravations that are a part of life. But did you know that stress is linked to weight gain?

Remember, when stress strikes, cortisol, the fight-or-flight hormone, is released, and the elevated cortisol levels make weight loss more difficult.[2]

But when you feel calm, centered, and relaxed, your body chemistry works for you instead of against you. Meet a remarkable, fast-working, shut-down-stress process that I call *The Cortisol-Calming Quickie.*

Diaphragmatic Breathing: The Key to Calm

The technique you're about to learn can help you immediately—and I mean *instantly*—calm down, anytime, anywhere. Whenever you feel tense, you'll quickly relax by doing *diaphragmatic breathing*, also known as belly breathing, deep breathing, or slow abdominal breathing.[3]

Think back to when you were anxious, and someone told you, "Just take a few breaths." There's a biological reason this works. When you take deep, slow breaths, you stimulate the vagus nerve. Also known as the vagal nerves, these are your parasympathetic nervous system's main nerves, which run from your brain through your face and thorax to your abdomen. They control your digestion, heart rate, and immune system.[4]

Before you invite calm in, you want to meet your diaphragm. This is the large, dome-shaped muscle located at the base of your lungs that separates your chest or thoracic cavity from your abdomen. Your abdominal muscles not only help to move your diaphragm, but they give you more power to empty your lungs.[5]

To do diaphragmatic breathing or belly breathing, you want to actively pull down your diaphragm with every breath you take. When you engage your diaphragm, stomach, and abdominal muscles, you're signaling your brain to slow your heart rate, lower your blood pressure, and decrease cortisol levels in your body.[6]

Here's how to do it:

- Place one hand on the middle of your upper chest and place the other hand on your stomach, beneath your rib cage but above the diaphragm.
- Slowly breathe in through your nose and draw your breath down toward your stomach.
- To exhale, tighten your abdominal muscles and let your stomach fall downward while you exhale through pursed lips. Your chest remains still.
- Repeat, taking four to six breaths a minute.[7]

That's diaphragmatic breathing. With practice, you won't need to use your hands to guide you.

Now, find out how I took belly breathing one step further.

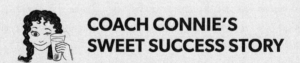

COACH CONNIE'S SWEET SUCCESS STORY

How I Created The Cortisol-Calming Quickie

My levels of stress were off the charts while I was with my mother in her dying months. While watching cancer take its brutal toll on Mom, I often needed to calm down—and fast.

One day, after my mother delivered that day's marching orders, I began to breathe deeply into my diaphragm while I inwardly told myself, "Peace of mind is mine now." Then, I slowly exhaled while again commanding myself, "Peace of mind is mine now."

Almost instantly, I felt soothed. Sure enough, I later found ample research to back up this easy tool, which will rapidly soothe, center, and relax you whenever you feel frazzled, edgy, or anxious.

THE PROOF:
The Fascinating Science about Diaphragmatic Breathing, the Basis of The Cortisol-Calming Quickie

Let's now look at some scientific studies about belly breathing's benefits:

- **Diaphragmatic breathing calms you down.** In a review of studies published in the *JBI Database of Systematic Reviews and Implementation Reports*, researchers found that diaphragmatic breathing significantly reduces measures of stress, including breathing rate, salivary cortisol levels, and blood pressure.[8]
- **When you do deep breathing, you may sleep better.** Research in *Frontiers in Psychiatry* observed that slow breathing "may be a more powerful tool in combating insomnia than the prevailing method of using hypnotics and other pharmaceutical interventions."[9] (Remember, sleeping sufficiently can help with weight loss.)
- **Diaphragmatic breathing may help burn more calories.** Scientists who examined two groups of people found that those who did diaphragmatic breathing had a significant increase in their resting metabolic rate (the measure of how many calories you burn) while the other group had none, the researchers pointed out in the *Journal of Physical Therapy Science*.[10]

> *The relaxation response is a physical state of deep rest that changes the physical and emotional responses to stress . . . and [is] opposite of the fight or flight response.*[11]
>
> **—Herbert Benson, MD** (1935–2022), author of *The Relaxation Response*, cardiologist, and founder of the Mind/Body Medical Institute at Massachusetts General Hospital in Boston

FEASTS (Fast, Easy, Awesome, Simple, Tested Strategies) to Self-Soothe with The Cortisol-Calming Quickie

Are you ready to calm down fast?

- **Do The Cortisol-Calming Quickie whenever stress strikes.** Take four to six slow deep belly breaths. During each inhale, count to five and think, "Peace of Mind is Mine Now." Then exhale to the count of five while you silently affirm, "Peace of Mind is Mine Now." Repeat for one to two minutes or more. Use this simple practice anywhere—while you run errands, wait for your kids, or rush to meet a deadline. No one will know what you're doing, and you'll feel better after just a few breaths.

- **If you get cravings, do The Cortisol-Calming Quickie.** If junk foods tempt you, this technique will shut down your cravings, redirect your energy, and bring on tranquility.
- **Chill out at night with The Cortisol-Calming Quickie.** This tactic helps if you feel anxious, have a lot on your mind, or wake up in the middle of the night.

Whenever you feel tense, just use this simple, science-based technique to claim calm, stay focused, and get peace of mind.

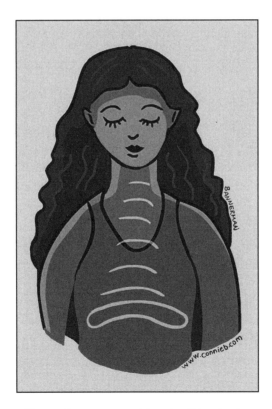

Discover the peace you get from breathing deeply
into your diaphragm, anytime... anywhere.

DAY 16

SUPERCHARGE WITH 21 POWER FOODS

*Choose your food wisely. Approach each meal as a chance to
enjoy something you truly value that is good for your health.
You have only so many meals left in your lifetime, so make each one
meaningful... Eat with the intent to improve your health.*[1]

—William W. Li, MD, president and medical director of the
Angiogenesis Foundation and *New York Times* bestselling author of
Eat to Beat Disease and *Eat to Beat Your Diet*

Now that you're eating real foods, you want to learn about some of the
awesome nutrients you're getting when you eat 21 Power Foods on the
Bounce Back Diet. These nutritious dynamos contain many helpful ingredients, including *antioxidants*, compounds that help prevent damage
caused by *free radicals* (molecules linked to aging and illnesses).

THE PROOF:
The Fascinating Science About 21 Power Foods

1. **Apple cider vinegar:** This has shown promise to improve
   insulin sensitivity and help lower blood sugar responses after
   meals. Studies have found that apple cider vinegar can be effective in reducing glucose and insulin levels after eating. It also
   may help shave off pounds.[2]

2. **Avocado:** This Power Food is a fruit (not a veggie) that is rich in
   monounsaturated fats, which may reduce "bad" low-density lipoprotein cholesterol in the blood and raise levels of the "good"
   high-density lipoprotein cholesterol. Avocados are high in vitamin E, which is important for your skin, brain, and immune
   system, and potassium, a mineral that helps your heartbeat stay
   regular, your muscles contract, and your nerves function.[3]

3. **Berries:** Yummy blueberries, blackberries, raspberries, and
   strawberries top the list of antioxidant-rich foods. Regularly eating berries (in modest portions, of course) can enhance immune
   function and reduce the kind of cellular inflammation that is
   associated with aging and chronic disease.[4]

4. **Black pepper:** This "King of Spices" is rich in a potent antioxidant called *piperine*, which may help prevent free radical damage, provide anti-inflammatory effects, and increase the absorption of various nutrients. Research shows that black pepper also may improve digestion, offer antimicrobial activity, and enhance fat metabolism.[5]

5. **Cacao (nibs or powder):** Cacao, which comes from the cacao bean, is really good for you *before* it's mixed with milk, cream, sugar, corn syrup, soy lecithin, palm oil, and other artificial or natural flavors to create unhealthy candy bars. Unsweetened cacao beans or nibs are great sources of fiber. Cacao also contains magnesium, which can help you relax and sleep better. Make sure to consume cacao earlier in the day, because it has some naturally occurring caffeine, which can keep you up.[6]

6. **Cinnamon:** This popular spice has anti-inflammatory and antioxidant qualities. Research suggests that as little as half a teaspoon a day of cinnamon may cut cholesterol and curb blood sugar by reducing insulin resistance.[7]

7. **Citrus Fruits:** Lemons, limes, and oranges are rich in immune-strengthening antioxidants and vitamin C.[8]

8. **Coconut oil:** Consuming the healthy medium-chain triglycerides (MCTS) found in coconut oil can induce modest weight loss without negatively impacting blood lipid levels.[9]

9. **Cruciferous vegetables:** Broccoli, Brussels sprouts, cabbage, cauliflower, collard greens, kale, kohlrabi, mustard greens, radishes, and turnips are all cruciferous vegetables, which provide fiber, vitamins, and phytochemicals (biologically active compounds in veggies).[10]

10. **Eggs:** Long shunned for being too high in cholesterol, "eggs now seem to be making a bit of comeback," according to the T. H. Chan School of Public Health. A study that looked at nearly 40,000 men and over 80,000 women suggests that moderate egg consumption of up to one a day "is not associated with increased heart disease in healthy individuals." Yolks contain most of an egg's protein and seven essential minerals, including

iron, potassium, and zinc. In addition, the protein in eggs helps you feel satiated.[11]

11. **Ginger:** This remarkable spice adds zing to your food, and ginger's main antioxidant, gingerol, has a host of health perks. For instance, ginger was found to improve digestive health, according to a review in *Nutrients*.[12]

12. **Garlic:** This much touted vegetable has anti-obesity properties. Research shows that supplementing the diet with garlic appears to reduce waist circumference.[13]

13. **Green Tea:** Research shows that green tea's catechins (phytochemical compounds) may help break down excess fat and increase fat burning. Although one cup of green tea contains less caffeine (about twenty-four to forty mg) as opposed to a cup of coffee (100 to 200 mg), it still can give you a mild buzz, so don't drink it six hours or less before bedtime. Or enjoy decaf green tea.[14]

14. **Leafy Greens:** Dark leafy greens such as arugula, bok choy (Chinese chard), broccoli rabe, collard greens, dandelion greens, kale, mustard greens, and Swiss chard are packed with fiber, vitamins, and minerals. They also contain nitrates, compounds that have been linked to a number of health benefits, including boosting your athletic performance.[15]

15. **Nuts: Almonds** have the most filling fiber of any nut, and research shows that snacking on them may reduce your overall calorie intake.[16] **Macadamia nuts** are rich in vitamins and minerals. They also have a moderately high fiber content, contain healthy monounsaturated fats, and can moderate your blood sugar levels.[17] **Pistachios** are a good source of protein, fiber, and antioxidants. Research found that 1.5 ounces of pistachios a day may help with weight loss.[18] **Pecans** are low in carbs (four grams per ounce), and one study found that a 1.5-ounce serving of pecans a day may offer protection against cardiovascular disease and type 2 diabetes.[19] **Pine nuts** (which aren't technically nuts but the seeds of pine trees) include healthy fats, filling fiber, and protein.[20] They also contain magnesium, which may help with glucose control. **Walnuts** may help activate the inula, the

part of the brain that regulates appetite and impulse control.[21] Remember that nuts are calorie-dense (a quarter-cup contains more than 200 calories), so portion control is crucial.

Know Your Allergies or Sensitivities

Before you consume the 21 Power Foods, please consult your health care provider to find out if you're allergic or sensitive to them. Please note that peanuts are the most common food allergy in the United States.[22]

16. **Olive oil:** This is superrich in monounsaturated fatty acids, which may help lower your "bad" LDL cholesterol and reduce body fat. One study found that those who consumed olive oil lost around 80 percent more body fat than those who used soybean oil.[23]

17. **Onions:** In addition to being a great low-calorie way to add flavor to foods, onions are rich in fiber. They're also low-glycemic, which means they don't have a significant impact on your blood glucose levels. Adding onions to your diet may help blunt blood sugar spikes that can trigger appetite.[24]

18. **Salmon:** Research suggests that this protein-rich seafood may increase your metabolic rate, reduce your appetite, increase insulin sensitivity, promote fat loss, and decrease belly fat in overweight people. Salmon is also packed with brain-and-heart-healthy omega-3 fats. If you can, get wild fresh or canned salmon instead of farmed salmon, which may contain toxins such as dioxins and PCBs.[25]

19. **Seeds:** Seeds are great sources of antioxidants, which may help reduce inflammation and regulate your immune system. **Chia seeds** are high in fiber and a good source of omega-3, a fat healthy for your heart.[26] **Flax seeds** are rich in omega-3s and a great source of lignans (part of the family of plant chemicals

known as polyphenols) and are linked to a reduced risk of breast cancer.[27] **Hemp seeds** are full of protein, omega-3s, vitamin E, and minerals.[28] **Pumpkin seeds** contain ample amounts of magnesium, which you need for strong bones and proper muscle contraction; zinc, which is important for immunity; and tryptophan, which can help promote sleep. Pumpkin seeds also may help maintain blood sugar control.[29] **Sesame seeds** contain ample calcium and vitamin E.[30]

20. **Sweet potatoes or yams:** These orange tubers contain fewer calories and carbs than white potatoes, and they pack plenty of fiber and protein. They're a good source of resistant starch, a substance that acts like fiber. Sweet potatoes and yams may lower the risk of obesity by helping prevent fat accumulation, enhancing insulin sensitivity, and regulating blood glucose levels and lipid metabolism.[31]

21. **Turmeric:** This bold yellow spice contains curcumin, an anti-inflammatory powerhouse. Research suggests that curcumin intake is linked to a reduction in weight, BMI, and waist circumference among patients with metabolic syndrome and related disorders.[32]

FEASTS (Fast, Easy, Awesome, Simple, Tested Strategies) to Enjoy Power Foods

You're already eating all 21 Power Foods on the Bounce Back Diet. Here are more ways to consume them:

- **Add Power Foods to meals.** To make salads, entrées, or vegetable dishes tastier and more nutritious, top them off with a teaspoon of ground flaxseed, pumpkin seeds, sesame seeds, and/or olive oil.
- **Season with Power Foods.** Boost the flavor and nutrition of your meals by adding apple cider vinegar, black pepper, garlic, ginger, onion, and/or turmeric.
- **Stash a healthy snack.** Keep small packets of premeasured, portion-controlled nuts, seeds, or nut butter in your car or desk drawer.

Bon appétit!

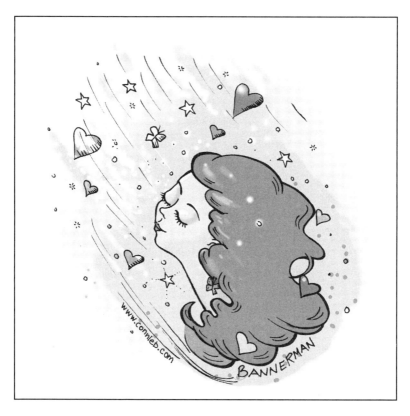

Shower yourself with self-compassion and forgiveness.

DAY 17

SHOWER YOURSELF WITH SELF-COMPASSION AND FORGIVENESS

A moment of self-compassion can change your entire day.
A string of such moments can change the course of your life [1]

—**Christopher K. Germer, PhD**, clinical psychologist
and author of the *Mindful Path to Self-Compassion:*
Freeing Yourself from Destructive Thoughts and Emotions

Today, we'll delve into two easy, scientifically validated practices—self-compassion and forgiveness—which will help you become more self-loving and accepting of yourself and others.

Let's start with compassion, which means "to suffer together."[2] Researchers consider compassion the feelings that come up when you see the suffering of others, and you feel motivated to relieve it. Self-compassion is when you're warm, understanding, and kind to yourself no matter what, even when you feel bad about any of your past perceived personal failings.[3]

Leading researcher Kristin Neff, PhD, an associate professor at the University of Texas at Austin and author of *Self-Compassion: The Proven Power of Being Kind to Yourself*, believes that self-compassion is "one of the most powerful sources of coping and resilience."[4]

However, it's often misunderstood. "One of the biggest myths about self-compassion is that it means feeling sorry for yourself," Dr. Neff explains. Quite the opposite. It is "an *antidote* to self-pity and the tendency to whine about our bad luck."[5]

I've been searching for ways to heal myself,
and I've found that kindness is the best way.[6]

—**Lady Gaga**, singer and songwriter

THE PROOF:
The Fascinating Science about Self-Compassion

Studies show that self-compassion ramps up your motivation; boosts happiness, self-confidence, and optimism; reduces anxiety, depression, and stress; diminishes your fear of failure; greatly lowers your desire for perfection; makes you feel more curious, creative, and grateful; increases your life satisfaction; cranks up your personal initiative, curiosity, and conscientiousness; enhances your self-worth; lessens body shame; and improves your self-image.[7] Consider these promising findings:

- **When you're self-compassionate, you accept your body.** In one compelling study, researchers found that self-compassion can help improve your body image. As the scientists explained in *Mindfulness*, participants listened to a twenty-minute self-compassion meditation daily for three weeks. Unlike those who relied only on self-control, subjects who tuned into self-compassion reduced their feelings of body shame and body dissatisfaction. Those improvements persisted during a three-month follow-up.[8]

- **If you write self-compassionate letters to yourself, you may feel better about your body.** A study in *Healthcare* suggested that a compassionate letter-writing exercise can help improve negative body image for females of all sizes. In addition, results indicate that penning compassionate words to yourself may affect levels of weight bias internalization (when you internalize society's negative stigma against those with higher BMIs).[9]

View your life with KINDSIGHT. Stop beating yourself up about things from your past. Instead of slapping your forehead and asking, "What was I thinking," breathe and ask yourself the kinder question, "What was I learning?"[10]

—**Karen Salmansohn,** bestselling author of *How to be Happy Damnit* and *Bounce Back! How to Thrive in the Face of Adversity*

THE PROOF:
The Fascinating Science about Forgiveness

Let's move on to a related topic—forgiveness. You may be wondering what releasing grievances has to do with the fact that you blew your diet. Actually, a lot.

Research cites a connection between not forgiving and eating badly. On the other hand, if you favor forgiveness, chances are better that you'll have a brighter outlook. In addition, when you cut yourself and others some slack, you may lessen your desire to use food to self-soothe.

When you let go of toxic anger, "your muscles relax, you're less anxious, you have more energy, [and] your immune system can strengthen," observes Robert Enright, PhD, author of *Forgiveness is a Choice*.[11]

Now, let me set the record straight: Forgiveness does *not* mean that you need to reconcile with those who've wronged you. You don't need to ever hang out with them again. But when you forgive others, you free up space to move on and become a healthier, happier person. Letting go of resentment is for your benefit, not theirs.[12]

> *Recasting your story is one of the keys of breaking free from the past.*
> *We must abandon the victim narrative and become our own protagonist.*[13]
> **—Katherine Schwarzenegger Pratt,** *New York Times*
> bestselling author of *The Gift of Forgiveness: Inspiring Stories*
> *from Those Who Have Overcome the Unforgivable*

You can find ample research about the benefits of forgiving:

- **When you practice forgiveness, you'll feel and sleep better.** Scientists, who surveyed more than 1,400 American adults, suggested in *Psychology & Health* that forgiving both others and yourself "may attenuate [reduce] emotions such as anger, regret, and rumination." That leads to "a restful mental state that supports sound sleep that, in turn, is associated with better health."[14]
- **Forgiveness knocks out stress.** For another study, participants were asked to "think of how you have responded to a person who has wronged or mistreated you." They also were asked to rate how strongly they agreed with statements such as, "I wish for good things to happen to the person who wronged me." Their responses were recorded on a measurement tool called the Rye Forgiveness Scale. The results, published in the *Annals of Behavioral Medicine*, indicate that "greater forgiveness is associated with less stress, and, in turn, better health."[15]
- **Self-forgiveness helps women eat better.** Letting go of resentment and anger benefitted women diagnosed with an eating disorder. Investigators from Walden University in Minneapolis found that those with an eating disorder possessed lower levels of self-forgiveness than women with normal dietary habits, according to a study in *Eating Disorders*.[16]

When you forgive, you heal your own anger and hurt and are able to let love lead again. [Forgiveness is] like spring cleaning for your heart.[17]

—**Marci Shimoff,** transformational teacher, author of the *New York Times* bestseller *Happy for No Reason*, and coauthor of the *Chicken Soup for the Woman's Soul*

How to Forgive with Ho'oponopono

Wondering how to forgive? Let me introduce you to the easy Hawaiian practice of Ho'oponopono, which means to "make it right" or "correct an error."

To do this technique, bring to mind a person or people who has/have wronged you. Then repeat the following four statements out loud or in your mind:

I'm sorry. Please forgive me. Thank you. I love you.

If this seems an unlikely way to forgive, don't take my word for it. Just try it and see if you make a shift.

You can learn more about Ho'oponopono in the fascinating book *Zero Limits: The Secret Hawaiian System for Wealth, Health, Peace and More*, by therapist Ihaleakala Hew Len, PhD and Joe Vitale.[18]

FEASTS (Fast, Easy, Awesome, Simple, Tested Strategies) to Shower Yourself with Self-Compassion and Forgiveness

- **Talk compassionately to yourself.** Try, *"Oh, [your name], it's okay that you blew your diet when [fill in the blank]. I love myself anyway, and I give myself the self-compassion I need."*
- **Comfort yourself with the Hug–Hum–Rock Relief Process.** Remember, that's one of the FEASTS that can bring you quick relief. To refresh your memory, see Day 8.[19]

- **Write yourself a self-compassionate letter.** This is your chance to speak kindly to yourself. Jot down words of praise, encouragement, and acceptance to lift yourself up.
- **Make a forgiveness list.** Write down names of people who've wronged you, living or dead, and then absolve them one by one using Ho'oponopono. Make sure to pardon yourself for any "stupid" things you said or did. Of course, also forgive yourself because you blew your diet.
- **Give yourself mirror love.** The late motivational guru Louise Hay touted the value of doing *mirror work*. Whenever you pass your reflection, speak compassionately to your image. "Doing mirror work is one of the most loving gifts you can give yourself," she advised. "It takes only a second to say, *"Hi, kid,"* or *"Looking good,"* or *"Isn't this fun?"* Go for it now! Find a mirror, affectionally hold your gaze, smile at yourself, and say, *I love you.*[20]
- **Create an Uplifting Mantra.** Here's an example: *"I forgive myself for everything I've done to hurt myself and others."*
- **Play forgiveness songs.** To deepen your experience, listen to tunes that put you in a merciful mood. Here are some ideas: "Forgiven" by contemporary Christian singer/songwriter David Crowder [21]; "Avinu Malkeinu" (Hebrew for "Our Father, Our King"), a hauntingly beautiful Jewish atonement prayer sung by Barbra Streisand[22]; "Forgive Me" by Evanescence[23]; "Sorry" by Ciara[24], and "Please Forgive Me" by Bryan Adams.[25]

By now, I hope, you feel psychologically lighter thanks to the power of practicing both self-compassion and forgiveness.

DAY 18

RELEASE YOUR SHAME
AND BOOST YOUR BODY IMAGE

If we base our self-worth on something as ever-changing as our bodies, we will forever be on the emotional roller coaster of body obsession and shame.[1]

—**Chrissy King**, writer, fitness and strength coach, and creator of The Body Liberation Project

You're now ready to face and triumph over any residual shame you may still have because you treated your body badly.

The late, renowned psychiatrist and psychoanalyst Carl Jung, MD, offered one of the best ways to address this emotion: "I want you to speak about your shame," he urged.[2]

Those of us who've felt trapped in *Weight-Gain Shameland* can tell you that it's a frustrating limbo, where you may be subjected to a litany of painful rejections, derisive insults, or callous putdowns from both others and from yourself. Yes, especially from you.

Sadly, people tend to shame others or themselves into shedding weight to *look* better, not to *feel* or *be* better. Focusing only on your appearance is the wrong way to approach weight loss.

To face shame head on, we turn to University of Houston research professor Brené Brown, PhD, who has studied shame, vulnerability, courage, and authenticity for more than a decade. She describes shame as "the intensely painful feeling or experience of believing that we are flawed and therefore unworthy of love and belonging."[3]

In her research, Dr. Brown, the *New York Times* bestselling author of such books as *Daring Greatly* and *Rising Strong*, found that body shame "is so powerful and often so deeply rooted in our psyche."[4]

Not only that, but its long reach "can impact who and how we love, work, parent, communicate and build relationships."

The good news, Dr. Brown contends, is that talking about shame blunts its power.[5]

"If we can share our story with someone who responds with empathy and understanding, shame can't survive."

Bounce Back Boldly Weight Success Story

I was spending so much mental energy just caught up in this body image and all the things I didn't like about myself. So I made a vow at that point that I would do whatever it took to . . . stop being critical of my body.

And I found this quote that made me really cry: "I said to my body for the first time, 'I want to be your friend,' and my body replied, 'I've been waiting my whole life for this.'" [That] just made me realize I had been fighting my body and shaming this amazing thing, the only body I'm ever going to get, trying to force it into submission. When really all it took was learning to take a deep breath and work with it versus always fighting."[6]

—**Katie Wells**, aka "Wellness Mama," an online source for naturally minded moms

THE PROOF:
The Fascinating Science About Fat Shaming

Studies show that negative talk backfires:

- **Fat shaming makes people gain** *more weight.* Researchers reviewing data from nearly 3,000 normal, overweight, and obese men and women found that those who experienced "weight discrimination" were *more likely* to have gained weight and increased their waist circumference during the four-year study period. As the scientists revealed in the journal *Obesity,* "weight discrimination [when people are excluded or treated in an inferior way] promotes weight gain and the onset of obesity."[7]

- **Loved ones bully or tease someone close to them the most.** One of the saddest findings I uncovered while researching this book is that close family members may say horrible things to their loved ones about their weight, according to a study in *Obesity*. When researchers from the Rudd Center for Food Policy and Obesity at Yale University asked nearly 2,500 overweight and obese adult men and women aged eighteen to eighty-nine "who stigmatized them the most," *a staggering 72 percent* of the subjects reported that family members were "the most judgmental or derogatory."[8]

▪ **Weight shaming leads to more weight gain and worse health.** In an opinion article in *BMC Medicine*, leading psychologists and sociologists observed that when overweight people felt that they experienced weight stigma, their "eating increases, their self-regulation decreases, and their cortisol levels are higher relative to controls, particularly among those who are or perceive themselves to be overweight." (The World Obesity Federation classifies weight stigma as "discriminatory acts and ideologies targeted toward individuals because of their weight and size."[9])

I love that people come up to me and say: "Because you are comfortable in your skin, you have made me more comfortable in mine." That's the best compliment ever.[10]

—**Kelly Clarkson**, American singer-songwriter known for the dazzling tune, "Whole Lotta Woman"

MORE PROOF: Science-Based Ways to Let Go of Your Shame and Boost Your Body Image

Now let's turn to happier news. You can rise above fat-shaming and feel better about your body no matter its present size. Research shows that a variety of science-based tactics can help, especially ones you learned about earlier in the Bounce Back Boldly Plan. For instance:

▪ **Shame subsides when you write yourself a kind letter.** Remember the study that highlighted the benefits you get by writing yourself a self-compassionate letter? Similarly, other scientists explained in their study in the publication *Mindfulness* that students with high shame experienced "significant decreases in both global and external shame" when they wrote themselves a self-compassionate letter.[11]

- **Journaling can help you better understand why you feel shame or guilt.** Writing about your thoughts or emotions for twenty minutes a day for three to four days brings clarity and relief. In fact, one study in *Psychological Science* from self-expressive writing expert Dr. James Pennebaker had the apt title, "Writing about Emotional Experiences as a Therapeutic Process."[12]
- **Writing can calm you down.** Writing about past failures can help you lower stress hormones such as cortisol, according to a study in *Frontiers in Behavioral Neuroscience*.[13]
- **Tapping may bring reductions in shame and other emotions.** Research found that the Emotional Freedom Technique can bring reductions in anxiety, depression, shame, PTSD, and other emotions. Tapping also can result in an increase in happiness.[14]
- **When you exercise, you may boost your body image.** If you do strength training twice a week for ten weeks, your body image and satisfaction may improve, according to a *Psychological Reports* study.[15] Meanwhile, for a study in *Body Image*, researchers found that women who exercised to calm down or feel better physically enjoyed greater improvements in their body image compared to those who exercised primarily for appearance reasons.[16]
- **You can retrain your brain to shun shame.** You may have heard the expression "neurons that fire together, wire together." This often-repeated phrase—which neuropsychologist Donald Hebb first used in 1949—refers to how we form pathways in our brains and then reinforce them through repetition. This is called *neuroplasticity*, which is when the brain can change and adapt due to input and experiences. To explain this simply, whenever you have a thought, feeling, or behavior that you'd like to repeat, you want to keep doing it. If, on the other hand, you have an unpleasant feeling such as shame in response to stimuli, your brain learns that response and it becomes harder to change. The good news is that when you train yourself to think kinder thoughts and be more self-compassionate, you can break the circuit and put in place more positive patterns.[17]

If you put shame in a petri dish, it needs three ingredients to grow exponentially: secrecy, silence, and judgment. If you put the same amount of shame in the petri dish and douse it with empathy, it can't survive.[18]

—**Brené Brown**, shame expert and author of *Daring Greatly*

FEASTS (Fast, Easy, Awesome, Simple, Tested Strategies) to Release Your Weight-Gain Shame and Boost Your Body Image

You've already learned proven tools that can help you move away from shame and towards body acceptance. Here are some awesome tactics to bring you to this happier place:

- **Tap away your shame.** Remember, one of your best tools to address and release painful emotions is to do tapping or Emotional Freedom Technique. (See Day 6.)
- **Write about shame experiences.** Bear in mind that writing is another transformational tool. (See Day 11.)
- **Shower yourself with self-compassion.** Giving yourself self-compassion can greatly reduce body dissatisfaction and body shame, as well as increase self-worth and body appreciation.[19] (See Day 17.)
- **Hit pause.** If you start to criticize your body, quickly replace those toxic thoughts with positive ones.
- **Be grateful for your remarkable body.** Appreciate your legs, hips, and thighs that take you places. Feel happy for your back and spine that allow you to stand upright. Enjoy your incredible hands, which can click away at the keyboard, text your buddies, lift your groceries, embrace your honey, or pick up your young ones. Rejoice in your miraculous body that lets you breathe, blink, think, talk, listen, create, smile, laugh, dance, make love, and sleep. (See Day 10.)
- **Create and repeat Body Love Affirmations.** Ramp up your body approval by boldly declaring and repeating Body Love Affirmations so often that they become mantras. Here's one to repeat: "I love and appreciate my awesome body."

- **See a therapist.** You also may find it helpful to talk about feelings of shame with a qualified psychologist, psychiatrist, or counselor.
- **Switch doctors if you're unhappy with your current one.** The good news is that the medical community now officially supports people of all sizes. In fact, an expert panel of thirty-six members issued a consensus statement in 2020 that was signed by 100 international medical organizations that called for ending weight stigma.[20]
- **Hang out in safe online spaces.** Unfollow any social media influencers, unfriend unsupportive friends, and stay away from any websites that make you feel bad about yourself or your body.
- **Feel pride while you move your body more.** Set a fitness target. Pick a goal, such as a one-hour walk, a 5K bike ride, or a one-hour yoga class. Leave shame behind while you get in shape.
- **Place your hand on your heart.** If any frustrating feelings about your body start to surface, warmly touch your heart, and send yourself love, acceptance, and compassion.
- **Remember that true beauty comes from within.** "When you feel good about yourself and who you are, you carry yourself with a sense of confidence, self-acceptance, and openness that makes you beautiful," points out the National Eating Disorders Association (NEDA). "Beauty is a state of mind, not a state of your body."[21]

You're on the way to love, appreciate, and enjoy your wonderful body.

DAY 19

PRACTICE MINDFUL EATING

Mindful eating is about awareness. When you eat mindfully,
you slow down, pay attention to the food you're eating, and savor every bite.[1]

—**Susan Albers, PsyD**, mindfulness expert, psychologist at the
Cleveland Clinic, and bestselling author of *Hanger Management* and
Quit Comfort Eating

What do a Buddhist monk, a Harvard-trained scientist, and a meditation teacher have in common?

They all know about a technique known as mindful eating, which "means simply eating or drinking while being aware of each bite or sip," according to the late Zen master Thích Nhất Hạnh and nutrition expert Lilian Cheung, coauthors of the book *Savor: Mindful Eating, Mindful Life.*[2]

When you eat mindfully, you're not just nourishing your body; you're also feeding your soul and recharging your spirit.

A Closer Look at Mindful Eating

What exactly do I mean by mindful eating? It's when you notice your physical hunger and eat only when you're hungry; pay attention to what you're eating; engage your senses so you notice colors, aromas, and textures; take small bites, eat slowly, savor your food, and know when you've had enough—before you're full. You'll also make healthier food choices and eat with both attention and intention.[3]

Mindful eating grew out of the fact that most of us "go unconscious when we eat," observes meditation teacher Jan Chozen Bays, MD.[4]

With mindful eating, you "tune into what your taste buds are saying" and "you awaken your inner gourmet," explains mindful eating researcher Jean Kristeller, PhD, a psychology professor emeritus at Indiana State University.[5]

"Even normal eaters participating in brief mindful eating workshops are often startled to discover the impact of mindful awareness both on increasing initial enjoyment and then letting go of the need to eat more."

We take somewhere between 50 and 100 bites per day.
By the time a person is 50, they've eaten something like
55,000 meals and taken in the neighborhood of 2 million bites.
Nothing except for sex engages your senses in such an intimate
and direct way. [W]hen we shine the light of our inquiring mind on
eating, we see so easily the connection between body and mind.[6]

—**Barry Boyce**, editor in chief of www.Mindful.org, and
author of the article "A Mindful Eating Revolution"

THE PROOF:
The Fascinating Science About Mindful Eating

Science validates the benefits of mindful eating:

- **Mindful eating helps people shed weight and be more aware.** People practicing mindful eating lost weight and continued to shed weight, according to an analysis in *Current Obesity Reports*. Mindful eating also helped "participants gain awareness of their bodies, be more in tune with hunger and satiety, recognize external cues to eat, gain self-compassion, decrease food cravings, decrease problematic eating, and decrease reward-driven eating," according to Carolyn Dunn, PHD, RD, and her colleagues from North Carolina University.[7]

- **When you eat mindfully, you eat more slowly and lose more weight.** A six-year study of nearly 60,000 obese subjects with type 2 diabetes investigated what happens when individuals change their eating speed. Fast eaters who became slow eaters had a 42 percent lower rate of obesity than those who continued to eat quickly, concluded a study in *BMJ Open*. Slow eaters notice "feelings of satiety before an excessive amount of food is ingested," the researchers found.[8]

- **Attentive eating curbs snacking.** Meanwhile, a team of researchers instructed women to eat lunch while listening to either a recording that encouraged them to notice the food they were eating or an audiobook unrelated to food. The study, published in the *British Journal of Nutrition*, found that those who listened to the food-focused audio had a better recall of what they consumed and ate 30 percent less.[9]

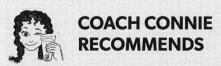

COACH CONNIE RECOMMENDS

Do Mindful Eating but Skip Sweets and Carbage

Although I'm a fan of mindful eating, I disagree with some of its principles. It's wrong, in my opinion, to tell people that they can mindfully eat *whatever they want* and that no foods are off limits.

As I shared previously, research found that eating ultra-processed foods can trigger a desire for more. Therefore, I urge you to eat mindfully while you also eliminate potentially addictive substances such as sugar, white flour, and all sweeteners.

To get the most out of mindful eating, I recommend that you mindfully eat *only* healthy, wholesome, nutrient-rich, clean foods that will enhance your moods, improve your concentration, and help you shed extra pounds.

FEASTS (Fast, Easy, Awesome, Simple, Tested Strategies) to be a Mindful Eater

- **Choose superior foods.** Carefully select high-quality foods to put into your wonderful body. On the Bounce Back Diet, you're doing just that.
- **Pay attention to the food in front of you.** Eat without distractions. Turn off the TV. Put away your phone. Notice how foods look, smell, and taste.
- **Give thanks.** Appreciate your food before you bite down and while you chew.
- **Dine.** Savor your food rather than bolt it down. Take in the "different aromas, textures, and tastes of everything you eat, instead of going from bite to bite—or, more often, swallow to swallow," recommends clinical neuropsychologist, mindfulness-meditation practitioner Jennifer Wolkin, PhD, author of *Quick Calm*.[10]

When you become more mindful, your enjoyment of food and appreciation of life will be magnified big-time.

DAY 20

USE YOUR FORMER "FAILURES" TO FUEL YOUR FUTURE SUCCESS

Failure is not fatal, it's just a necessary stepping stone to success.
Embrace it, learn from it, and use it to bounce back stronger than ever before![1]

—**Barbara Corcoran**, investor, entrepreneur, and former *Shark Tank* star,
who had straight Ds in school and twenty jobs by age twenty-three

Now that you're well on your way to a healthier, happier life, you're strong
enough to think about your former "failures" around food. Most importantly, you need to know that no matter how many times you abandoned
a healthy way of eating in the past, you are *not* a failure now.

Rather, your former mistakes mean that you're getting *much closer* to
success. Those hurdles can help intensify your commitment and determination to succeed and ensure your resilience.

Do not be embarrassed by your failures,
learn from them and start again.[2]

—**Richard Branson**, British business magnate
and founder of the Virgin Group

Inspiring People "Failed" Their Way to Spectacular Success

History is full of inventors, authors, actors, and entrepreneurs who tried,
failed, and then ultimately succeeded, often wildly. Let these persistent
people motivate you:

- Long before **Thomas Edison** invented the light bulb, phono-
  graph, and motion picture camera, he was considered by teachers
  "too stupid to learn anything." The innovator insisted that "failure
  is success in progress. I have not failed," Edison said. "I've just
  found 10,000 ways that won't work."[3]
- Long before author **J. K. Rowling** wrote the biggest bestselling
  book series in history, she was an unemployed, depressed, single
  mother living in a cramped apartment with her daughter. Then she

was fired from a secretarial job for daydreaming too much. (She was secretly spinning stories on her work computer.) Later, the aspiring author received twelve rejections from publishers for her first *Harry Potter* book. At press time, fans worldwide had snapped up more than 500 million copies of Rowling's *Harry Potter* novels.[4]

- Long before **Oprah Winfrey** became host of the most successful TV talk show in history, a media mogul, actress, philanthropist, bestselling author, and one of the world's richest women, she was fired from a news reporter job in Baltimore. Her higher-ups considered her "unfit for TV news" and "too emotionally invested" in her stories. Those traits, of course, helped lead to the success of *The Oprah Winfrey Show*, which ran for twenty-five seasons. "You learn the most about yourself when you appear to fail," Oprah said. "Every time a crisis or disruption comes, it's here to teach me or wake me up or make me sharper."[5]

- Long before **Steven Spielberg** became the force behind such creative blockbusters as *Jaws*, *Close Encounters of the Third Kind*, *E.T. The Extra-Terrestrial*, *The Color Purple*, and *Schindler's List*, he got poor grades in high school and was rejected three times by the University of Southern California's film school.[6]

- Long before **Tyler Perry** became a prolific writer, producer, actor, and creator of the popular "Madea" character, he was a struggling, homeless playwright living in his car. Now, he owns the 330-acre, Atlanta-based Tyler Perry Studios, the nation's largest film production studio.[7]

- And long before **Lisa Nichols** became a *New York Times* bestselling author and top motivational speaker, she was fired from five jobs and told by a teacher that she should never do public speaking. "I believe that all of my successes today are because I failed at something in the past and pulled the best lessons out. The power lies in getting back up," contends Nichols.[8]

These are just a few examples of super-successful people, who weren't deterred by perceived failures.

You only get to success when you're willing to fail along the way.[9]

—**Kerry Washington**, actress and former *Scandal* star, who was interviewing Reese Witherspoon while guest-hosting *Jimmy Kimmel Live*

Failures Can Be Springboards to Success

Of course, failure can be painful. Even so, "it actually can allow us to unlock great potential," observed award-winning scientist Anna Powers, PhD.[10]

"Instead of seeing [failure] as something detrimental to success, we have to see it as a tool for success, a tool that helps us refine our path and allows us to learn what works and what does not," Dr. Powers wrote in an article for *Forbes*.

"In such a way, we can see it as a normal part of the innovation of our own lives, not as something detrimental to life."

> *If we look backward with the specific intent of moving forward, we can convert our regrets into fuel for progress. They can propel us toward smarter choices, higher performance, and greater meaning.*[11]
>
> **—Daniel Pink**, *New York Times* bestselling author of *The Power of Regret: How Looking Backward Moves Us Forward*

THE PROOF: The Fascinating Science about How Failure is a Stepping Stone to Success

Now let's look at some enlightening studies about failure:

- **Early failures can lead to future success.** A study in *Nature* from Northwestern University's Kellogg School of Management looked at the career success of nearly 140,000 young scientists who *narrowly missed* getting grants from the National Institutes of Health, compared to those who *narrowly won* them. The scientists who were denied grants had *more successful* publications in academic journals *five years later* than those who received grants.[12]
- **Learning about scientists' difficulties improves students' likelihood of success.** After 400 high school students found out about personal and intellectual struggles of renowned scientists Albert Einstein and Marie Curie, their science grades *improved*. However, students who learned *only* about the scientists' achievements

scored *lower grades*, according to a study published in the *Journal of Educational Psychology*.[13]

- **Successful athletes cite setbacks as instrumental to their success.** UK scientists looked at the traits of fifty-six European athletes competing in soccer, rugby, rowing, curling, shooting, skiing, karate, judo, and boxing. These top-tier athletes spoke about how their setbacks, injuries, or getting cut from a team became *catalysts* rather than *roadblocks*, according to a study in *Frontiers in Psychology*. When faced by challenges, those high achievers became *more driven to succeed*. In discussing an injury, one "super champion" said, "It just kicked me where it hurt, and I was determined to get back." Another athlete, who didn't make the "selection, especially after all that work" decided, "I was never ever going to let them beat me. I just did double everything!"[14]

Surrender to what is. Let go of what was. Have faith in what will be.[15]

—**Sonia Ricotti**, personal transformation expert and bestselling author of *Unsinkable: How to Bounce Back Quickly When Life Knocks You Down*

FEASTS (Fast, Easy, Awesome, Simple, Tested Strategies) to View Your Diet "Failures" as a Great Opportunity to Become Healthy

Let's relate this discussion of failure to your situation:
- **Reframe what brought you here.** Starting today, use your former setbacks to become *more determined* to eat better.
- **Let your previous "failures" teach you the value of persistence.** Realize that your former flops have helped you develop the stellar traits of tenacity, grit, and resilience.
- **Consider your former "failures" as the start of something wonderful.** Because you ate badly in the past, you can now rewrite your future so you have a healthier weight and life.

You've now learned from super-successful people who once "failed." Like they did, let your repeated "failures" become stepping stones to your success.

DAY 21

LET NATURE NURTURE YOU

*I understood at a very early age that in nature, I felt everything
I should feel in church but never did. Walking in the woods, I felt
in touch with the universe and with the spirit of the universe.*[1]

—**Alice Walker**, novelist, poet, activist, and author of
the Pulitzer Prize-winning novel *The Color Purple*

When was the last time you were out in Mother Nature where you watched swallows soar or squirrels scurry, inhaled the scent of fragrant azaleas and tulips, and listened to seagulls squawk or cicadas buzz?

It's time to get outdoors to revel in stunning natural wonders. Now, if you're like most people, you'll associate being outdoors with exercising, but you don't need to break a sweat to derive benefits.

*Short exposures to nature can make us less aggressive,
more creative, more civic minded and healthier overall.*[2]

—**Florence Williams**, journalist and author of *The Nature Fix:
Why Nature Makes Us Happier, Healthier, and More Creative*

THE PROOF: The Fascinating Science About How Mother Nature Nurtures Us

Ample evidence confirms what nature lovers have long known—that exposure to natural environments, from parks to woodlands to beaches, is calming, restorative, and linked to better health. For instance:

- **Nature reduces stress.** More than 19,000 people who spent two hours a week in nature experienced "increases in good health and wellbeing," according to a survey published in *Scientific Reports*.[3]
- **As little as ten minutes in nature boosts moods.** College students who sat or walked in nature for ten to twenty minutes experienced beneficial effects on their mental health, pointed out a study in *Frontiers in Psychology*.[4]
- **Living close to green areas lowers the risk of gaining weight.** A study in the *International Journal of Hygiene and Environ-*

mental Health—which examined data from nearly 2,400 female city dwellers in Spain for five years—found that those who lived within 300 meters (about 1,000 feet) from parks, trails, or green spaces in urban settings had a *decreased* risk of being overweight or obese.[5]

- **"Forest bathing" makes you happier and healthier.** Mindfully immersing yourself in wooded areas or doing the Japanese practice of forest bathing (*shinrin-yoku*) by using all five senses is beneficial in many ways. For instance, research shows that spending time in nature may reduce stress, anxiety, depression, confusion, and anger; boost the immune system; improve cardiovascular and metabolic health; and lead to increased feelings of "awe."[6] Forest bathing also may provide a preventive effect on cancers and improve sleep, according to Japanese doctor and researcher Qing Li, MD, PhD, professor at Tokyo's Nippon Medical School, an expert in forest medicine, and author of the book *Forest Bathing: How Trees Can Help You Find Health and Happiness.*[7]

MORE PROOF: Nature's Remarkable Fractals

Now let me introduce you to miraculous fractals. These are the "fingerprints of nature" that you find in leaves, trees, branches, ferns, mountains, ocean waves, snowflakes, seashells, rocks, sand dunes, rivers, terrains, coastlines, and clouds. (They're also in crystals, cauliflower, and Romanesco broccoli.) Fractals are one reason you feel so darn good in nature. Consider:

- **Watching fractal patterns in nature reduces stress levels by up to 60 percent.** "The effects of fractals are almost instantaneous," University of Oregon physicist and fractals expert Richard Taylor, PhD, explained to me. "Your visual system is in some way hardwired to understand fractals. The stress reduction is triggered by a physiological resonance that occurs when the fractal structure of the eye matches that of the fractal image being viewed."[8]
- **Just sixty seconds in nature can increase people's alpha brain waves.** Researchers measured the brain waves of people while watching nature's wonders and found that seeing fractals *for as little as one minute* led to changes in their alpha brain waves, according to a study from Dr. Taylor that was published in *Nonlinear Dynamics, Psychology, and Life Sciences.*[9] (Alpha brain waves are

known for their ability to reduce anxiety, boost creative thinking, lower stress, decrease depression, and increase pain tolerance.)[10]

Nature Can Nurture You While You're Indoors, Too

If your schedule is too hectic or the weather foul, Mother Nature can still nurture you when you're indoors:

- **Listening to nature sounds and watching natural scenes brings benefits.** As they explained in *Scientific Reports*, researchers who measured people's brain activity using an MRI scanner concluded that listening to five-minute, twenty-five-second recordings from nature helped individuals relax and lowered their heart rates. Those who listened to artificial sounds reacted like people suffering from anxiety, PTSD, or depression.[11]
- **Looking at photos of nature helps lower stress levels.** Watching pictures of green areas for *only five minutes* may help people recover from stress, according to research in the *International Journal of Environmental Research and Public Health*. Images of buildings and parked cars didn't have that soothing effect.[12]
- **Watching plants is beneficial.** Even taking care of indoor plants can reduce physiological and psychological stress, according to research in the *Journal of Physiological Anthropology*.[13]

FEASTS (Fast, Easy, Awesome, Simple, Tested Strategies) to Let Nature Nurture You

Here are some tips to enjoy nature's wonders:

- **If you feel stressed, get outside for fifteen minutes.** Go for a walk. Watch the majesty of a tree. Listen to birds singing. Marvel at cloud formations.
- **Aim for awe.** Lose yourself in a sunset. Enjoy the changing colors, lights, and shadows. In short, relish Mother Nature's magnificence.
- **Focus on fractals.** While outdoors, appreciate those repeating, complex patterns in trees, ferns, and flowers.
- **Layer your benefits.** Take a walk or yoga class in the park at sunrise or sunset. Go for a bike ride on tree-lined streets.

- **Bring nature home.** If you can't get outside, try these:
  - ☐ Watch videos of waves crashing against the shore. The color blue fosters calm and creativity. Plus, the rhythmic swelling and cresting of waves has a healing, hypnotic effect.
  - ☐ Watch YouTube videos of chirping forest birds and mesmerizing waterfalls.
  - ☐ Hang nature photos on the walls of your office and home.
  - ☐ Start an herb or vegetable garden on your windowsill or in your yard.
  - ☐ Collect seashells, rocks, or crystals.
  - ☐ Pick or buy sweet-smelling flowers, and place them in a pretty vase where you can enjoy them often.

You're Bouncing Back Boldly! It's Dance Party Time

Woo Hoo! You did it! You completed the Bounce Back Boldly Plan. You should be so proud of yourself. You're on your way to having an amazing life.

To continue receiving benefits and shed more weight, keep practicing those FEASTS that most resonated with you. Make them a part of your everyday life.

Now you want to rejoice alone or with loved ones. Of course, we're having another Dance Party. Put on your favorite comfy clothes and sneakers. Clear an area in your home.

Now stand up, sway, and let loose to these invigorating songs while you continue to Bounce Back Boldly:

- "Brave" by Sara Bareilles[14]
- "Fix You" by Coldplay[15]
- "Good Times Roll" by Jimmie Allen[16]
- "Better in Time" by Leona Lewis[17]
- "Nothing's Gonna Stop Us Now" by Starship[18]

While you happily dance, take pride in all that you've accomplished and confidently celebrate the fact that you're on your way to becoming the happier, healthier, awesome person you know you can be.

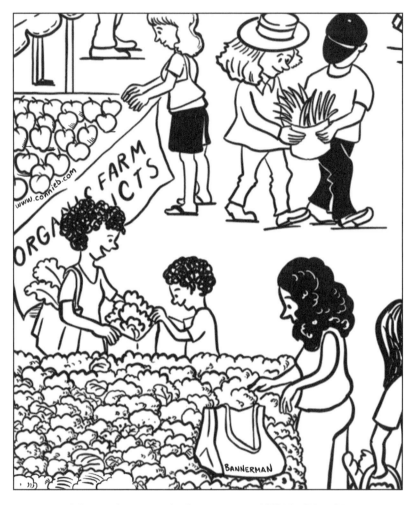

If there's a farmers market in your area, go ASAP! You'll love it!

Part IV

What to Eat

The
Bounce Back
Diet

Recipes and Meal Plans
Developed by Lizette and Geoff Marx

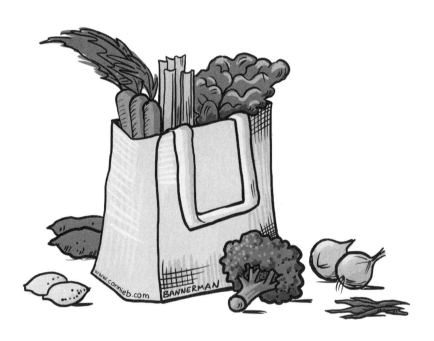

Chapter 22

Shopping Lists
and Meal Plans

*Tell me what you eat and
I will tell you who you are.*[1]
—**Jean Anthelme Brillat-Savarin** (1755–1822),
French epicure, lawyer, politician,
and author of *Physiology of Taste*

It's now my pleasure to present the Bounce Back Diet, a clean, nutrient-dense, modified ketogenic (KetoMod) way of eating. This is a less restrictive, more realistic, low-carb, anti-inflammatory plan that's plentiful in healthy fats, quality protein, and real carbs.

All recipes and meal plans for the 21-day Bounce Back Diet were lovingly developed by the talented chefs Lizette and Geoff Marx, who created tasty dishes that will help you shed excess weight and overhaul your relationship with food.

You'll shed pounds, because every day you'll consume ample protein (75 to 90 grams), fat (90 to 100 grams), nonstarchy carbs (40 grams or less), and fiber (30 grams or more).[2] Because you're cutting carbs and eating enough protein and fat, the pounds will slide off as you retrain your metabolism to burn fat and build muscle.

The Bounce Back Diet's delicious dishes are intended to awaken your taste buds and help you easily transition to a cleaner, healthier way of eating without sacrificing flavor. On this KetoMod plan, you'll boost your consumption of fiber, protein, and quality fats. In addition, you'll use organic herbs and spices.

On the Bounce Back Diet, you'll prepare nutrient-rich, appetizing, energy-dense meals with vegetables, nuts, seeds, superfoods, lean meats, seafood, bone broth, seasonings, healthy fats, and small amounts of low-sugar fruits.

In addition, several times a week, you'll enjoy our grounding Bounce Back Golden Milk, refreshing Bounce Back Chia Fresca, and soothing Bountiful Bone Broth.

You'll never be hungry on the Bounce Back Diet, because you'll never go longer than three hours between meals or snacks, except, of course, between dinner and breakfast the next morning. This way your blood sugar levels will always remain stable.

While you eat better, you'll avoid gluten, dairy, and all caloric sweeteners, including agave, barley malt, brown rice syrup, cane sugar, cane syrup, coconut sap, coconut sugar, date sugar, monk fruit, and honey. In addition, you'll eliminate artificial sweeteners and sugar alcohols such as xylitol and erythritol. You'll also stay away from soy products other than miso, which is naturally fermented and an easy-to-digest source of minerals and enzymes.

At the end of each week, you'll get one serving of a lip-smacking, nutrient-dense, clean KetoMod dessert. These end-of-meal treats are so yummy that you'll wonder how they can contain no sugar, sweeteners, dairy, gluten, or artificial sweeteners.

Your Staple Ingredients Shopping List

You'll now find a list of nonperishable pantry items that will last the entire three weeks of the Bounce Back Diet. We've specified certain brands that we trust for their high quality.

Oils/Vinegars/Condiments

- Apple cider vinegar, 1 (10-fluid ounce) bottle, Bragg
- Avocado oil, 1 (32-ounce) bottle
- Capers, 1 (2-ounce) jar
- Champagne vinegar, 1 (10-fluid ounce) bottle
- Coconut oil, unrefined, 1 (14-ounce) jar
- Coconut butter, 1 (14-ounce) jar
- Dijon mustard, 1 (4-ounce) jar
- Extra-virgin olive oil, 3 (32-ounce) bottles
- Ghee, 2 (9-ounce) jars
- Ginger juice, unsweetened, 1 (5-ounce) bottle
- Gomasio, 1 (3.5-ounce) jar, Eden Foods
- Green olives, pitted, 5 (10.2-ounce) jars
- Horseradish paste, 1 (9-ounce) jar
- Kalamata olives, pitted, 3 (10.2-ounce) jars
- Kombu seaweed, 1 (1.75-ounce) package
- Lemon juice, 100 percent pure, 1 (12-fluid ounce) bottle
- Liquid Aminos, sugar-free, 1 (16-fluid ounce) container, Bragg
- Miso paste, 1 (9-ounce) container
- Mayonnaise, sugar-free, 1 (12-ounce) bottle, Primal Kitchen Mayo
- Rice vinegar, 1 (10-fluid ounce) bottle
- Sesame oil, toasted, 1 (8-fluid ounce) bottle

Nuts and Seeds

- Almond butter, 1 (16-ounce) jar
- Almonds, dry-roasted (no salt), 1 (16-ounce) pouch or bag
- Cashews, 2 (16-ounce) pouches or bags
- Chia seeds, 1 (8-ounce) pouch or bag
- Flaxseed meal or ground flaxseed, 1 (1-pound) bag or container
- Pecans, 2 (16-ounce) pouches or bags
- Pistachios (dry-roasted), 1 (24-ounce) pouch or bag
- Pepitas or no-shell pumpkin seeds, 1 (12-ounce) pouch or bag
- Tahini, 1 (16-ounce) jar
- Walnuts, 2 (16-ounce) pouches or bags

Baking/Spices

- Almond flour, 5 (1-pound) bags
- Baking soda, 1 (8-ounce) box
- Bay leaf, whole, 1 (.15-ounce) jar
- Black pepper, ground or whole black peppercorns, 1 (1.80-ounce) jar
- Cardamom, ground, 1 (1.87-ounce) jar
- Cayenne pepper, ground, 1 (1.87-ounce) jar
- Chili flakes, 1 (1.87-ounce) jar
- Chili powder, 1 (1.87-ounce) jar
- Cinnamon, ground, 1 (1.87-ounce) jar
- Coconut flakes or shredded coconut, unsweetened, 1 (7-ounce) pouch
- Coriander, ground, 1 (1.87-ounce) jar
- Cumin, ground, 1 (1.87-ounce) jar
- Curry, ground, 1 (1.87-ounce) jar
- Garam masala, 1 (2-ounce) jar
- Garlic powder, 1 (2.4-ounce) jar
- Ginger, ground, 1 (1.52-ounce) jar
- Himalayan sea salt, fine ground, 1 (8-ounce) jar
- Italian seasoning, 2 (0.95-ounce) jars
- Oregano, 2 (0.36-ounce) jars
- Paprika, 1 (1.87-ounce) jar
- Thyme, 1 (0.63-ounce) jar
- Turmeric, ground, 1 (1.92-ounce) jar
- Vanilla, alcohol-free, 1 (4-fluid ounce) jar
- Vanilla bean, 2 beans in a jar or package
- White pepper, 1 (0.45-ounce) jar or package
- Za'atar spice, 1 (1.5-ounce) jar

Canned/Boxed/Other

- Almond milk, unsweetened, 2 (32-fluid ounce) cartons
- Cashew milk, unsweetened, 2 (32-fluid ounce) cartons
- Chicken bone broth or stock, organic, sugar-free, unsalted/sea salt, 8 (32-fluid ounce) cartons, packages, or frozen containers.
- Coconut milk, unsweetened, full-fat, BPA-free, 5 (13.66-fluid ounce) cans, Native Forest or Organic Thai Kitchen
- Meat sticks (beef, turkey, or chicken), 13 (1.7-ounce), Nick's Sticks
- Salmon, vacuum-sealed, flash frozen
- Shirataki (konjac) noodles, 2 (7-ounce) packages, Miracle Noodle

- Tomatoes, diced, organic, BPA-free can, 3 (14.5-ounce) cans
- Vegetable stock, organic, sugar-free, sea salt only or unsalted, 4 (32-fluid ounce) cartons
- Wild, line-caught albacore tuna, 2 (5-ounce) cans, Wild Planet

Staples And Brands We Like[3]

You can get quality, often-organic, usually pesticide-free foods from the websites listed below. These companies make some or all of their products without sweeteners or artificial sweeteners, but please read ingredients lists before you buy anything to verify that the formulations haven't changed:

- Annie's Organics, www.annies.com
- Artisana, www.artisanaorganics.com
- Bragg (Liquid Aminos) www.Bragg.com
- Butcher Box, www.butcherbox.com
- Califia Farms, www.califiafarms.com
- Carrington Farms, www.carringtonfarms.com
- Chosen Foods, www.chosenfoods.com
- Eden Foods, www.store.edenfoods.com
- Frontier Co-Op, www.frontiercoop.com
- Garden of Life, www.gardenoflife.com
- Miracle Noodles, www.miraclenoodle.com
- Nick's Sticks, www.nicks-sticks.com
- Organic Valley, www.organicvalley.coop
- Pacific Foods, www.pacificfoods.com
- Primal Kitchen, www.primalkitchen.com
- Santa Cruz Organic, www.santacruzorganic.com
- Sea 2 Table, www.sea2table.com
- Simply Organic, www.simplyorganic.com
- Spectrum Organics, www.spectrumorganics.com
- Vital Choice, www.vitalchoice.com
- Wild Alaska Salmon & Seafood Company www.wildalaskasalmonandseafood.com
- Wildly Organic, www.wildlyorganic.com
- Wild Planet, www.wildplanetfoods.com

Herbal Teas

- Adagio Teas, www.adagio.com
- Art of Tea, www.artoftea.com
- Good Earth, www.goodearth.com
- Organic India, www.organicindia.com
- Traditional Medicinals, www.traditionalmedicinals.com
- Tazo, www.tazo.com
- Yogi Tea, www.yogitea.com

In addition to finding all staples for the Bounce Back Meal Plan at the websites cited above, you can purchase them from your local grocery store, health food supermarket, or from their websites. Here are a few popular places to shop:

www.Albertsons.com	www.Ralphs.com
www.Amazon.com	www.Safeway.com
www.Costco.com	www.Sprouts.com
www.iHerb.com	www.Target.com
www.Kroger.com	www.TraderJoes.com
www.LuckyVitamin.com	www.ThriveMarket.com
www.PigglyWiggly.com	www.Vitacost.com
www.Publix.com	www.WholeFoods.com

Look at our farmers' markets today, bursting with heritage breeds and heirloom varieties, foods that were once abundant when we were an agricultural nation, but that we have lost touch with. Bringing all these back helps us connect to our roots, our communities, and helps us feed America the proper way.[4]

—**José Andrés**, culinary innovator, one of *Time's* "100 Most Influential People," and founder of World Central Kitchen

Buy From Local Farmers

While you stock up on groceries, buy the best quality produce and protein you can find. Here are ways to do that:

- **Go to a farmers' market.** If your area has a weekly farmers' market, start going. The friendly, knowledgeable, health-conscious vendors—who raised the foods they sell—usually avoid pesticides. Just ask. (Insecticides or fungicides can cause a number of adverse reactions.[5]) All vendors sell food they've grown locally, within a few hours' drive away. This means that the foods you buy are tastier, healthier, and fresher. Plus, veggies, fruits, eggs, chicken, beef, meats, flowers, and other products likely cost far less than in grocery stores. To find a farmers' market near you, enter your zip code into the USDA's directory: www.ams.usda.gov/local-food-directories/farmersmarkets.[6]

- **Join a CSA.** Another option to find quality foods is to join a nearby Community-Supported Agriculture, or CSA. Members get reasonably priced, weekly, full or half shares of seasonal, locally sourced veggies, eggs, meats, poultry, fruit, flowers, and herbs from a specific farm or group of farms in your region. www.localharvest.org/csa/.[7]
- **Purchase unusual-shaped real foods.** You also can buy excess, different-shaped, healthy foods that are rescued before they're ditched into landfills for being "ugly."
  - ¤ **Imperfect Foods** delivers affordable, high-quality "imperfect" groceries, which may have "cosmetic quirks, irregular sizes, or are just surplus." www.imperfectfoods.com[8]
  - ¤ **Misfits Market** also delivers organic produce and high-quality meats and seafood at up to 40 percent off grocery store prices. www.misfitsmarket.com[9]

Real food doesn't have ingredients.
Real food is the ingredients.[10]

—Jamie Oliver, British restaurateur
and bestselling author of *7 Ways* and *5 Ingredients*

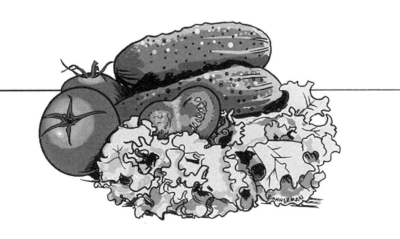

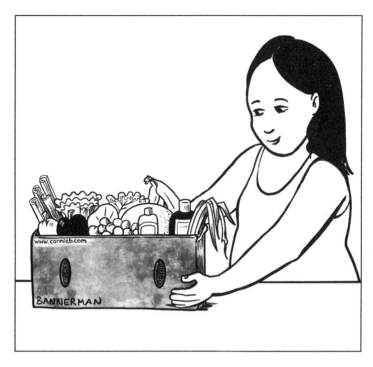

"I love having healthy foods and staples shipped directly to me."

Beyond-the-Book Support:
Get My List of Healthy Snacks to Pack

Now that you're on your way to eating cleanly, always be prepared. Whenever you leave home, always keep blood-sugar balanced foods handy. For ideas on what to bring with you when you're on the go, get my Healthy Snacks to Pack list. Access it at at <u>www.ConnieB.com/Healthy-Snacks-to-Pack</u>.

WEEK 1 Grocery Shopping List

Produce

- 5 medium onions
- 3 small onions
- 1 small red onion
- 8 shallots
- 3 garlic heads
- 1 jalapeño
- 4 red bell peppers
- 3 cucumbers
- 1 small claw, fresh ginger
- 1 fresh turmeric root (1-inch piece)
- 1 bunch radishes
- 2 bunches basil (or enough for 2 cups tightly packed leaves)
- 5 green onions
- 1 bunch dill
- 1 bunch tarragon, optional
- 1 small bunch oregano
- 1 bunch Italian flat-leaf parsley
- 2 bunches cilantro
- 1 bunch celery
- 1 medium leek
- 2 carrots
- 5 medium zucchinis
- 1 medium spaghetti squash
- 3 bunches baby bok choy greens
- 3 bunches broccolini or broccoli
- 3 medium fennel bulbs
- 1 large head cauliflower
- 1 head of escarole or collard greens
- 4 large bunches kale
- 3 bunches rainbow chard
- 1 (5-ounce) box baby arugula or other dark leafy greens
- 2 small heads or 2 (7-ounce) boxes Romaine hearts or baby gem lettuce
- 2 (7-ounce) boxes Romaine hearts or 1 head Romaine lettuce
- 1 head butter lettuce
- 1 medium head green globe cabbage
- 1 small head purple cabbage
- 1½ pounds shiitake mushrooms
- 2 (1-pint) containers cherry tomatoes
- 3 medium red tomatoes (Roma or vine-ripened)
- 3 avocados (Haas if available)
- 1 Granny Smith or other tart green apple
- 1 pomegranate
- 1 (6-ounce) container raspberries
- 6 lemons or 1 (10-fluid ounce) bottle 100 percent lemon juice (no sugar or additives)

- 4 limes or 1 (10-fluid ounce) bottle 100 percent lemon juice (no sugar or additives)

Refrigerated Dairy Alternatives
- 1 (8-ounce) container unsweetened cashew, almond, or coconut yogurt

Meat and Eggs
- 2 dozen large eggs
- 1 whole, cooked rotisserie chicken (seasoned with herbs and spices only)
- 4 pounds chicken bones
- 4 boneless, skinless chicken breasts
- 6 skin-on, bone-in chicken thighs
- 2 pounds ground turkey thigh
- 1¼ pounds skirt or flank steak
- 1 package turkey bacon
- 1 pound beef stew meat
- 1 pound king or coho salmon fillet
- ½ pound crab meat

Recipes to Prep for Week 1
To save time, make the following recipes a day or two before you start the Bounce Back Diet:
- Bounce Back Chia Fresca
- Bounce Back Golden Milk
- Dazzling Dijon Shallot Dressing
- Marinate the Golden Power Skirt Steak on Day 5
- Bountiful Bone Broth (This recipe makes 5 quarts, enough to last the three-week plan.)

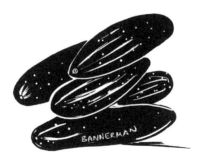

WEEK 1 Meal Plan

DAY 1

Morning Balance Beverage
Bounce Back Chia Fresca

Breakfast
1 slice of **As-You-Like-It Frittata** and 1½ cups of arugula tossed in 1 tablespoon of **Dazzling Dijon Shallot Dressing**

Snack
1 (8-ounce) mug of **Bountiful Bone Broth** and 1 slice of toasted **Olive Rosemary Nut-Flax Focaccia** with 1 teaspoon of ghee

Lunch
Win-Win Turkey-BLT Salad with Avocado Lime Dressing

Snack
1 **Zucchini Spice Muffin** or 1 meat stick (Nick's Sticks) with ¼ cup raspberries

Dinner
Pound-it-Out Chicken Cutlets with Cilantro Pepita Verde Sauce
Served on a bed of zucchini or shirataki noodles

DAY 2

Morning Balance Beverage
Bounce Back Chia Fresca

Breakfast
1 slice of toasted **Olive Rosemary Nut-Flax Focaccia** with smashed avocado, chopped hard-boiled egg, and a pinch each of Himalayan sea salt and smoked paprika

Snack
½ cup of sliced cucumber topped with Himalayan sea salt, a squeeze of fresh lemon juice, and 3 walnuts

Lunch

Grateful Herb Garden Salad tossed with leftover **Cilantro Pepita Verde Sauce** and chopped leftover **Pound-It-Out Chicken Cutlets**

Snack

1 (8-ounce) mug of **Bounce Back Golden Milk** and 1 **Zucchini Spice Muffin**

Dinner

Wild Roasted Salmon with Mustard Horseradish Butter and **Stir-Fried Broccolini and Bok Choy with Crispy Shiitake Mushrooms**

DAY 3

Morning Balance Beverage
Bounce Back Chia Fresca

Breakfast

1 slice of leftover **As-You-Like-It Frittata** and 1½ cups of arugula tossed in 1 tablespoon of **Dazzling Dijon Shallot Dressing**

Snack

1 (8-ounce) mug of **Bountiful Bone Broth** with a squeeze of lemon, if desired, and 1 **Zucchini Spice Muffin**

Lunch

Leftover **Stir-Fried Broccolini and Bok Choy with Crispy Shiitake Mushrooms** with leftover **Wild Roasted Salmon with Mustard Horseradish Butter**

Snack

½ cucumber sliced and ½ red bell pepper sliced, with ¼ cup **Zesty Lemon Pepper Zucchini Tahini Spread** to use as a dip or 1 of Nick's Sticks with ½ cup sliced cucumber and red pepper

Dinner

Crazy-Good Crab Cakes with **Garlic Aioli** and **Shred-Your-Stress Tahini Ginger Coleslaw**

DAY 4

Morning Balance Beverage
Bounce Back Chia Fresca

Breakfast
Leftover **Crazy-Good Crab Cakes** with 1 poached egg

Snack
1 (8-ounce) mug of **Bounce Back Golden Milk** or herbal tea of
  choice and 1 **Zucchini Spice Muffin**

Lunch
Grateful Herb Garden Salad with **Creamy-Better-for-You
  Ranch Dressing**

Snack
1 slice of toasted **Olive Rosemary Nut-Flax Focaccia** with
  2 tablespoons **Zesty Lemon Pepper Zucchini Tahini Spread**

Dinner
**Crispy Provençal Herb Chicken Thighs, Creamy-Dreamy
Cauliflower Mash**, and green salad with sliced cucumber and
tomatoes with **Creamy-Better-for-You Ranch Dressing**

DAY 5

Morning Balance Beverage
Bounce Back Chia Fresca

Breakfast
Sumptuous Seasonal Scrambled Eggs

Snack
1 (8-ounce) mug of **Bountiful Bone Broth** with a squeeze of
  lemon and a pinch of cayenne, if desired, and 1 **Zucchini Spice
  Muffin**

Lunch
1 leftover **Crispy Provençal Herb Chicken Thigh** with 1½ cups
  of arugula tossed in 1 tablespoon of **Dazzling Dijon Shallot
  Dressing** and **Creamy Cauliflower Soup**

Snack
½ avocado sprinkled with Himalayan sea salt and paprika and 1
  tablespoon of chopped dry roasted pistachios or 1 of Nick's Sticks

Dinner

4 **Herby Turkey Meatballs** with **Spaghetti Squash Noodles** and **Garlicky Basil Cream Sauce**

Healthy Nightcap

1 (8-ounce) mug of **Bounce Back Golden Milk**

DAY 6

Morning Balance Beverage

Bounce Back Chia Fresca

Breakfast

2 hard-boiled large eggs, chopped and served with 1 tablespoon of **Oh-So-Good Olive Walnut Tapenade**

Snack

½ tart green apple, sliced, with 1 tablespoon of unsweetened almond butter or 1 of Nick's Sticks

Lunch

Embrace-Your-Inner-Goddess Chopped Salad and 2 leftover **Herby Turkey Meatballs**

Snack

1 stalk of celery cut into 3 pieces or ½ red bell pepper cut into 3 wedges and filled with 1 tablespoon each of **Zesty Lemon Pepper Zucchini Tahini Spread**

Dinner

Golden Power Skirt Steak with **Feels-Like-I'm-Cheating Creamed Greens** and **Spicy Oven Cauli "Fries"**

DAY 7

Morning Balance Beverage

Bounce Back Chia Fresca

Breakfast

Sassy-Saucy Poached Eggs with Rainbow Chard

Snack

1 **Zucchini Spice Muffin** and a cup of herbal tea of choice

Lunch

Leftover **Embrace-Your-Inner-Goddess Chopped Salad** with leftover **Golden Power Skirt Steak** cut into strips and **Spicy Oven Cauli "Fries"**

Snack

½ avocado with a pinch of Himalayan sea salt, ⅛ teaspoon of fresh-squeezed lemon juice, and 1 tablespoon of pepitas or 1 of Nick's Sticks

Dinner

Better-Than-Mom's Chicken Soup with 1 **Get-Cozy Scallion Almond Biscuit** and a tossed mixed green salad with **Avocado Lime Dressing**

Dessert

2 **Chocolate Spice Coconut Crunch Truffles**

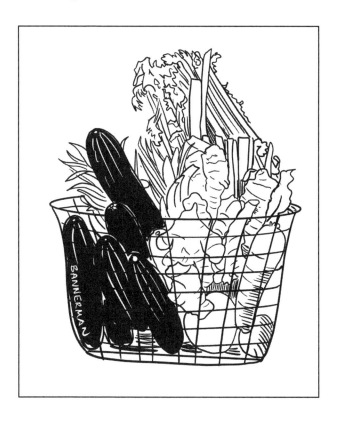

WEEK 2 Grocery Shopping List

Produce

- 1 large red onion
- 1 small red onion
- 5 medium yellow onions
- 8 shallots
- 3 garlic heads (24 cloves)
- 1 bunch scallions (green onions)
- 1 bunch celery
- 1 small claw ginger root
- 1 fresh turmeric root (1-inch piece)
- 1 jalapeño
- 6 lemons
- 4 limes
- 1 red tomato (Roma or vine-ripened)
- 2 (1-pint) containers cherry tomatoes
- 4 avocados (Haas or whatever is available)
- 2 English cucumbers
- 2 carrots
- 4 zucchinis
- 1 medium spaghetti squash
- 3 medium heads cauliflower
- 1 large celery root
- 1½ pounds green beans
- 5 red bell peppers

- 1 bunch asparagus
- 3 bunches broccolini or broccoli
- 3 bunches baby bok choy
- 1 small head red or green globe cabbage
- 1 bunch rainbow chard
- 5 bunches dark leafy greens (kale, chard, collard, or a mix of all three)
- 1 bunch lacinato (also called dinosaur) kale
- 1 bunch curly kale (green or purple)
- 1¼ pounds shiitake mushrooms
- ½ pound cremini mushrooms
- 3 bunches basil
- 1 bunch Italian flat-leaf parsley
- 1 bunch fresh dill
- 1 bunch fresh tarragon
- 1 small bunch fresh thyme
- 2 bunches cilantro
- 1 (2-ounce) package pea shoots
- 1 (5-ounce box) arugula
- 1 (8-ounce) box baby kale
- 1 pomegranate

Refrigerated Non-Dairy

- 1 (8-ounce) container, unsweetened cashew, almond, or coconut yogurt

Meat and Eggs

- 2 dozen large eggs
- 4 bone-in, skin-on chicken thighs
- 2 bone-in, skin-on chicken breasts
- 4 boneless, skinless chicken breasts
- 1¼ pounds skirt steak
- ½ pound turkey thigh meat
- ½ pound ground bison or beef
- 1 pound beef stew meat
- 4 (4-ounce) halibut fillets
- 1 (5-ounce) can tuna

Recipes to Prep for Week 2

To streamline your week, make these recipes in advance:

- Bounce Back Chia Fresca
- Bounce Back Golden Milk
- Bounce Back Bountiful Bone Broth, if needed
- Marinate the Healing Slow Roasted Chicken with Lemons, Olives, and Capers on Day 7
- Marinate the Golden Power Skirt Steak on Day 9

We need to become friends with food again. It's a relationship we need to spend time on and really invest in. When we go from obsessing about diet foods to eating foods that nourish us, from obsessing about losing weight to obsessing about learning how to thrive with better health, we enjoy the journey of discovering what is best for us.[11]

—**Jessica Ortner,** host of the Tapping World Summit and author of the *New York Times* bestselling book *The Tapping Solution for Weight Loss & Body Confidence*

WEEK 2 Meal Plan

DAY 8

Morning Balance Beverage
Bounce Back Chia Fresca

Breakfast
Leftover **Sassy-Saucy Poached Eggs with Rainbow Chard** with 1 warmed leftover **Get-Cozy Savory Scallion Almond Biscuit**

Snack
1 (8-ounce) mug of **Bountiful Bone Broth**

Lunch
Embrace-Your-Inner-Goddess Chopped Salad and a bowl of leftover **Better-Than-Mom's Chicken Soup**

Snack
1 **Zucchini Spice Muffin** or 1 of Nick's Sticks and a cup of herbal tea

Dinner
Healing Slow Roasted Chicken with Lemons, Olives and Capers, Cauliflower Couscous, and **Basil Arugula Pesto**

DAY 9

Morning Balance Beverage
Bounce Back Chia Fresca

Breakfast
Sumptuous Seasonal Scrambled Eggs

Snack
½ avocado with a pinch of Himalayan sea salt and paprika

Lunch
Oodles of Zoodles and Koodles with Almond Ginger Turmeric Dressing

Snack
1 (8-ounce) mug of **Bounce Back Golden Milk**

Dinner
Pistachio Crusted Halibut with 4 roasted asparagus spears
and 1 cup of **Spaghetti Squash Noodles**

DAY 10

Morning Balance Beverage
Bounce Back Chia Fresca

Breakfast
1 warmed leftover **Get-Cozy Savory Scallion Almond Biscuit**,
  topped with one poached egg,
3 tablespoons of **Silky Pecan Cream Sauce,** and 1 slice of tomato
  with a pinch of Himalayan sea salt

Snack
1 (8-ounce) mug of **Bountiful Bone Broth** and 1 **Zucchini Spice
Muffin** or 1 of Nick's Sticks

Lunch
2 cups of baby kale and arugula tossed with **Tahini Ginger
  Dressing** and leftover **Healing Slow Roasted Chicken**

Snack
½ cup sliced cucumber topped with a pinch of Himalayan sea salt,
  ¼ teaspoon of fresh-squeezed lemon juice, and 1 tablespoon of
  leftover **Oh-So-Good Olive Walnut Tapenade**

Dinner
Golden Power Skirt Steak and **Thyme-Scented Green Beans
with Chopped Almonds**

DAY 11

Morning Balance Beverage
Bounce Back Chia Fresca

Breakfast
1 poached egg on salad greens tossed with leftover **Thyme-Scented
  Green Beans**

Snack
1 (8-ounce) mug of **Bounce Back Golden Milk**

Lunch

Leftover **Golden Power Skirt Steak** cut into strips and served on a bed of spinach and arugula with ½ chopped avocado, toasted pepitas, and **Dazzling Dijon Shallot Dressing**

Snack

1 **Zucchini Spice Muffin** and a cup of rooibos chai or herbal tea of choice

Dinner

Wild Roasted Salmon (omit horseradish butter and use leftover **Almond Ginger Turmeric Dressing**) and **Stir-Fried Broccolini and Bok Choy with Crispy Shiitake Mushrooms**

DAY 12

Morning Balance Beverage
Bounce Back Chia Fresca

Breakfast

Leftover **Wild Roasted Salmon** and 1 warmed **Get-Cozy Savory Scallion Almond Biscuit**

Snack

1 (8-ounce) mug of **Bountiful Bone Broth** and 1 **Zucchini Spice Muffin** or 1 of Nick's Sticks

Lunch

Embrace-Your-Inner-Goddess Chopped Salad with 2 medium-boiled eggs sprinkled with Himalayan sea salt and a pinch of paprika

Snack

½ avocado with a sprinkle of Himalayan sea salt and paprika

Dinner

Moroccan Cottage Pie with **Need-to-Knead Kale Salad**

Soothing Nightcap
1 (8-ounce) mug of **Bounce Back Golden Milk**

DAY 13

Morning Balance Beverage
Bounce Back Chia Fresca

Breakfast
Sassy Saucy Poached Eggs with Rainbow Chard

Snack
½ cup sliced cucumber with a sprinkle of Himalayan sea salt with **Oh-So-Good Olive Walnut Tapenade** and 1 tablespoon of chopped almonds

Lunch
1 toasted slice of **Olive Rosemary Nut-Flax Foccacia** topped with 3 tablespoons of **Sunflower Avocado Tuna Spread** and leftover **Embrace-Your-Inner-Goddess Chopped Salad**

Snack
1 (8-ounce) mug of **Bountiful Bone Broth** or 1 **Zucchini Spice Muffin**

Dinner
Pound-It-Out Chicken Cutlets with **Cilantro Pepita Verde Sauce** and **Spicy Oven Cauli "Fries"**

DAY 14

Morning Balance Beverage
Bounce Back Chia Fresca

Breakfast
Feels-Like-I'm-Cheating Creamed Greens with 2 poached eggs and 1 slice of turkey bacon

Snack
½ cup sliced cucumber with a sprinkle of Himalayan sea salt, ¼ teaspoon of fresh-squeezed lemon juice, and 3 walnuts

Lunch
Leftover **Moroccan Cottage Pie** and **Grateful Herb Garden Salad** tossed with **Dazzling Dijon-Shallot Dressing**

Snack

3 **Kale Chip Krispies** with 1 slice of toasted **Olive Rosemary Nut-Flax Focaccia** with **Oh-So-Good Olive Walnut Tapenade** spread on top or 1 of Nick's Sticks

Dinner

Savory-and-Sublime Spicy Miso Beef Stew with **Oodles of Zoodles and Koodles** and **Almond Ginger Turmeric Dressing**

Dessert

2 **Lemon Coconut Cream Bon-Bons**

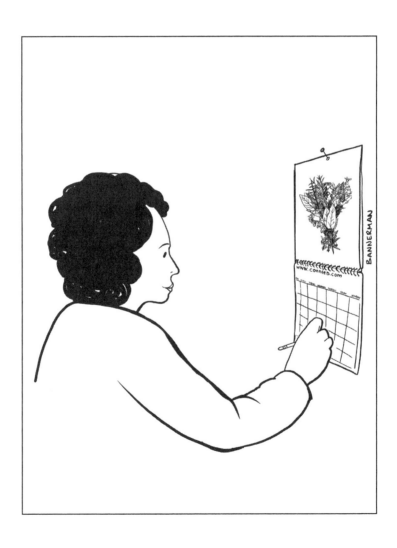

WEEK 3 Grocery Shopping List

Produce

- 1 large red onion
- 1 medium red onion
- 6 medium yellow onions
- 11 shallots
- 4 garlic heads
- 1 small claw ginger root
- 1 fresh turmeric root (1-inch piece)
- 1 jalapeño
- 1 bunch scallions (green onions)
- 3 cucumbers
- 3 zucchinis
- 1 bunch celery
- 2 red bell peppers
- 1 (1-pint) container cherry tomatoes
- 3 tomatoes (Roma or vine-ripened)
- 3 medium fennel bulbs
- 2 leeks
- 1 (3-pound) spaghetti squash
- 3 large cauliflower heads
- 1 large celery root
- 3 bunches dark leafy greens (chard, kale, escarole, or a mix of all three)
- 3 bunches lacinato (aka dinosaur) kale
- 1 bunch curly kale (green or purple)
- 1 bunch rainbow chard
- 1 pound Brussels sprouts
- 1 small green globe cabbage
- 1 small purple cabbage
- ½ pound cremini mushrooms
- 2 bunches basil
- 1 bunch thyme
- 1 bunch dill
- 1 bunch Italian flat-leaf parsley
- 1 bunch cilantro
- 1 (5-ounce) container baby arugula
- 1 (5-ounce) container baby spinach leaves
- 1 (10-ounce) container romaine hearts, butter lettuce, or baby gem lettuce
- 1 (4-ounce) container sprouts (your choice)
- 4 avocados (Haas or whatever is available)
- 8 lemons
- 3 limes
- 1 (6-ounce) container blueberries
- 1 (8-ounce) container raspberries
- 1 pomegranate
- 1 Granny Smith or other tart green apple

Refrigerated Non-Dairy
- 1 (8-ounce) container unsweetened cashew, almond, or coconut yogurt

Meat and Eggs
- 3 dozen eggs + 4
- 1 whole, cooked rotisserie chicken (seasoned with herbs and spices only)
- 4 pounds chicken bones, backs, necks, and wings
- 6 skin-on, bone-in chicken thighs
- 1 (8-ounce) package turkey bacon
- 2½ pounds ground turkey thigh
- ½ pound ground bison or beef
- 1¼ pounds skirt steak
- 1 pound king or coho salmon fillet
- 4 (4-ounce) halibut fillets
- 1 (5-ounce) can tuna

Recipes to Prep for Week 3
To streamline your week, make the following recipes in advance:
- Bounce Back Chia Fresca
- Bounce Back Golden Milk
- Bountiful Bone Broth (Make more if you're running low.)

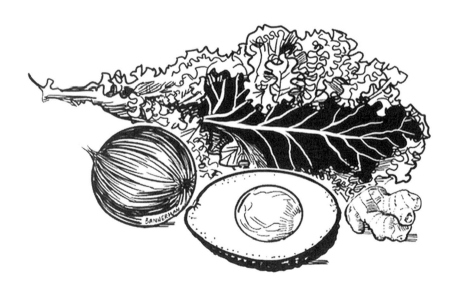

WEEK 3 Meal Plans

DAY 15

Morning Balance Beverage
Bounce Back Chia Fresca

Breakfast
Sumptuous Seasonal Scrambled Eggs with 1 slice of
  Olive Rosemary Nut-Flax Focaccia

Snack
1 (8-ounce) mug of **Bountiful Bone Broth** and 3 leftover
  Kale Chip Krispies or 1 of Nick's Sticks

Lunch
Shred-Your-Stress Tahini Ginger Coleslaw with leftover
  Savory-and-Sublime Spicy Miso Beef Stew

Snack
½ avocado with 1 tablespoon of sunflower seeds and a sprinkle of
  Himalayan sea salt and paprika

Dinner
Crispy Provençal Chicken Thighs, **Thyme-Scented
Green Beans** with **Chopped Almonds**, and **Creamy-Dreamy
Cauliflower Mash**

DAY 16

Morning Balance Beverage
Bounce Back Chia Fresca

Breakfast
As-You-Like-It Frittata

Snack
½ cup sliced cucumber and 1 piece of celery, cut into thirds with
  Creamy Better-for-You Ranch Dressing

Lunch
Leftover **Grateful Herb Garden Salad** with **Dazzling Dijon
  Shallot Dressing** and 1 **Crispy Provençal Chicken Thigh**

Snack

1 (8-ounce) mug of **Bounce Back Golden Milk** or herbal tea of choice and 1 **Zucchini Spice Muffin**

Dinner

Pistachio Crusted Halibut and **Confetti Brussels Sprouts with Leeks and Turkey Bacon**

DAY 17

Morning Balance Beverage

Bounce Back Chia Fresca

Breakfast

1 poached egg on leftover **Confetti Brussels Sprouts with Leeks and Turkey Bacon**

Snack

1 (8-ounce) mug of **Bountiful Bone Broth** and/or 1 slice of toasted **Olive Rosemary Nut-Flax Focaccia** with ½ teaspoon of ghee

Lunch

2 baby gem, butter, or romaine lettuce cups filled with ⅓ cup each of **Sunflower Avocado Tuna Spread**

Snack

1 **Zucchini Spice Muffin** or 1 of Nick's Sticks and ¼ cup of raspberries or blueberries

Dinner

Herby Turkey Meatballs with **Cauliflower Couscous** topped with **Basil Arugula Pesto**

DAY 18

Morning Balance Beverage

Bounce Back Chia Fresca

Breakfast

1 leftover slice of **As-You-Like-It Frittata**

Snack
½ avocado with a sprinkle of Himalayan sea salt, ⅛ teaspoon of
fresh-squeezed lemon juice, and 1 tablespoon of chopped walnuts

Lunch
Leftover **Herby Turkey Meatballs** with **Embrace-Your-Inner-Goddess Chopped Salad**

Snack
1 (8-ounce) mug of **Bounce Back Golden Milk** and 1 **Zucchini Spice Muffin**

Dinner
Golden Power Skirt Steak with **Spaghetti Squash Noodles**
and **Almond Ginger Turmeric Dressing**

DAY 19

Morning Balance Beverage
Bounce Back Chia Fresca

Breakfast
Win-Win Turkey-BLT Salad with **Avocado Lime Dressing**
and 1 poached or chopped hard-boiled egg

Snack
1 (8-ounce) mug of **Bountiful Bone Broth**

Lunch
Shred-Your-Stress Tahini Ginger Coleslaw with leftover
Golden Power Skirt Steak

Snack
½ cup of cucumber slices with ¼ cup **Zesty Lemon Pepper
Zucchini Tahini Spread** or 1 of Nick's Sticks

Dinner
Sassy-Saucy Poached Eggs with Rainbow Chard and
1 **Get-Cozy Savory Scallion Almond Biscuit**

Soothing Nightcap
1 (8-ounce) mug **Bounce Back Golden Milk**

DAY 20

Morning Balance Beverage
Bounce Back Chia Fresca

Breakfast
1 **Get-Cozy Savory Scallion Almond Biscuit** with a green
salad with chopped avocado, sliced hard-boiled egg, broccoli or
sunflower sprouts, and **Dazzling Dijon-Shallot Dressing**

Snack
½ sliced apple with 1 tablespoon of almond butter

Lunch
Better-than-Mom's Chicken Soup

Snack
Kale Chip Krispies and ½ cup sliced cucumber with ¼ cup **Zesty
Lemon Pepper Zucchini Tahini Spread** or 1 of Nick's Sticks

Dinner
Moroccan Cottage Pie with **Need-to-Knead Kale Salad**

DAY 21

Morning Balance Beverage
Bounce Back Chia Fresca

Breakfast
Sumptuous Seasonal Scrambled Eggs and 1 warmed leftover
Get-Cozy Savory Scallion Almond Biscuit

Snack
½ cup sliced cucumber topped with a sprinkle of Himalayan sea salt,
¼ teaspoon of fresh-squeezed lemon juice, and 1 tablespoon of
chopped walnuts

Lunch
Grateful Herb Garden Salad with **Creamy-Better-for-You
Ranch Dressing** and leftover **Better-than-Mom's Chicken
Soup**

Snack
1 (8-ounce) mug of **Bounce Back Golden Milk** with ¼ cup
raspberries or blueberries

Dinner

Wild Roasted Salmon with **Mustard Horseradish Butter,**
    Spicy Oven Cauli "Fries," and **Shred-Your-Stress Tahini**
    Ginger Coleslaw

Dessert

Coconut Vanilla Panna Cotta with Toasted Coconut

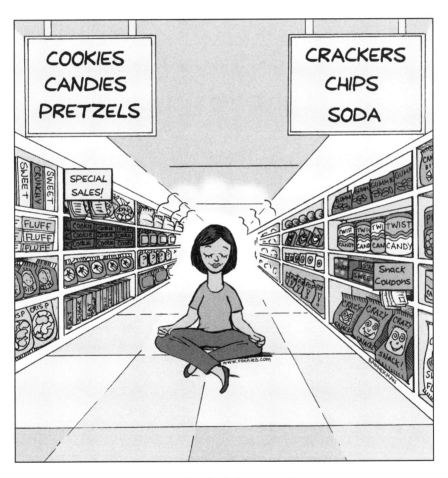

You can claim calm in the grocery store.

Chapter 23

The Bounce Back
Diet Recipes

*We believe that cooking from home is a healthy practice just like taking
a morning walk. Make meals a consistent ritual in your day, choose real
food, cook with love and mindfulness, and savor every delicious bite.*[1]

—Lizette and Geoff Marx, professional holistic chefs,
culinary nutrition consultants, and creators of the recipes and
meal plans on the Bounce Back Diet

It's time to enjoy real, nutritious, delicious foods. All recipes below are
listed alphabetically by category. Have fun in the kitchen making tasty
foods that will make your body feel good!

BEVERAGES

While you follow the Bounce Back Diet, you'll drink three healthy, flavorful, restorative beverages:

- **Bounce Back Chia Fresca** is our hydrating take on a Central and South American-inspired drink.[2] Fiber-rich chia seeds promote feelings of fullness, stabilize blood sugar levels, and support weight loss. Make sure to soak the seeds in filtered water for at least 20 to 30 minutes before using so they're easier to digest. Eating unsoaked chia seeds may cause bloating or stomach pain.[3] See page 258.

- Our **Bounce Back Golden Milk** was inspired by an Ayurvedic beverage popular in India. You can enjoy this unsweetened drink either warm or chilled. For the latter, pour it over ice or blend with ice cubes in a blender. Our recipe includes ground flaxseed, which is rich in soluble and insoluble fiber and gives this beverage a creamy texture.[4] See page 259.

- Finally, in between meals, you can sip our nutritious, flavorful, low-calorie **Bounce Back Bountiful Bone Broth**. You also can add it to recipes. If you prefer to buy it premade, you can purchase it from a variety of vendors. See page 270.

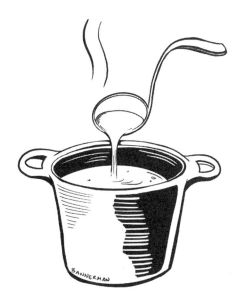

Bounce Back Chia Fresca

Yield: 1 quart

Serves 4 (8-ounce) glasses

Ingredients

1 quart filtered water, divided*

2 tea bags or 2 teaspoons of loose-leaf tea: ginger, lemon balm, peppermint, licorice, or your favorite herbal tea*

½ lemon, juiced

1 lime, juiced, optional

¼ teaspoon unsweetened ginger juice or ginger, powdered or ground to taste

1½ teaspoons chia seeds

Directions

- Boil 2 cups of water and remove from heat. Add the tea and steep for 10 minutes. Remove the tea bags and pour into a medium-sized, heat-proof jar with a tight-fitting lid. If you use loose leaf tea, set a strainer over the jar and pour tea through to catch the tea leaves. Discard the leaves. Stir in the remaining water, lemon and/or lime juice, ginger, and the chia seeds. The chia seeds may settle to the bottom, so stir occasionally to distribute the seeds or tighten the cap on the jar and give it a shake.

- Make sure to soak the chia seeds in the tea for at least 20 to 30 minutes before serving so they'll absorb water, become gelatinous, and be easier to digest. Keep the Bounce Back Chia Fresca in the fridge and enjoy every morning as your Morning Balance Beverage. If you like, you can drink it at room temperature. This also makes a great afternoon beverage.

CULINARY TERM: *When a recipe lists an ingredient followed by the word **divided**, this means that you'll use half earlier and the other half later.*

HEALTH TIDBIT: *All herbal teas have different health benefits.[5] For instance, you may choose teas that may boost your immune system, help with digestion, or calm your nervous system. See shopping list on page 231 for brands we like.*

Bounce Back Golden Milk

Yield: 1 quart
Serves 4 (8-ounce) mugs

Ingredients

2 cups unsweetened almond or cashew milk

1 can full-fat, unsweetened coconut milk

6 tablespoons coconut butter

¼ cup ground flaxseed

2 teaspoons ground turmeric

½ teaspoon ground ginger

1 teaspoon ground cinnamon

1 teaspoon vanilla powder, vanilla bean seeds, or vanilla extract, optional

1 teaspoon ground cardamom

1 teaspoon ground fennel (if you only have the seeds, use them)

½ teaspoon freshly cracked pepper

Pinch* of Himalayan sea salt

Directions

- Add all ingredients to a blender and blend until smooth. Heat one serving (8 ounces) at a time in a saucepan over low heat until hot for a warm, soothing, delicious, immune-boosting, anti-inflammatory beverage.

- Store the remaining Bounce Back Golden Milk in a Mason jar or other airtight container and refrigerate. This soothing tonic will thicken when stored in the fridge so when you reheat it, just stir in a little water to thin the beverage to your desired consistency.

 CULINARY TERM: *A* **pinch**[6] *is about ¹⁄₁₆ of a teaspoon. When cooking, grab the salt between your thumb and index finger for a pinch. To get a better feel for how much this is, use half of a ⅛ teaspoon.*

What is really important . . . is to [ask yourself]:
"How do I feel when I eat this food?"[7]

—**JJ Virgin**, certified nutrition specialist, exercise physiologist, and *New York Times* bestselling author of *The Virgin Diet* and others

SALADS

Embrace-Your-Inner-Goddess Chopped Salad
Serves 4

Ingredients

2 cups chopped tomato (about 4 medium tomatoes)

1 cup chopped cucumber

1 cup chopped zucchini

1 small red bell pepper, chopped

1/3 cup fresh basil leaves, cut into ribbons

1/2 cup chopped, pitted black olives

1/2 tablespoon extra-virgin olive oil

1/2 tablespoon champagne vinegar or apple cider vinegar

1/4 teaspoon Himalayan sea salt

1/8 teaspoon freshly cracked black pepper

Directions

- Prepare all ingredients and toss together in a bowl. Season to taste with Himalayan sea salt and freshly cracked pepper. Chill before serving.

Grateful Herb Garden Salad
Serves 2

Ingredients

3 cups greens (butter lettuce or romaine hearts)

3 cups baby spinach, kale, or arugula

1/2 cup cherry tomatoes, sliced

1 small cucumber, sliced into rounds

1 watermelon radish or 2 red radishes, thinly sliced

1/4 cup chopped basil leaves

2 tablespoons chopped dill

2 tablespoons chopped, fresh Italian flat-leaf parsley

2 tablespoons sunflower seed kernels, toasted

Directions

- Toss all ingredients together with salad dressing of choice in a large bowl. Choose from *Tahini Ginger Dressing, Avocado Lime Dressing, Almond Ginger Turmeric Dressing, Creamy Better-for-You Ranch Dressing*, or *Dazzling Dijon-Shallot Dressing*.

Need-to-Knead Kale Salad

Serves 6

Ingredients

3 medium shallots, thinly sliced

½ cup extra-virgin olive oil, divided

½ teaspoon Himalayan sea salt, divided

3 garlic cloves, smashed

1 lemon, juiced

2 teaspoons Dijon mustard

⅛ teaspoon freshly cracked black pepper

2 bunches kale (lacinato or dinosaur), stems removed, leaves cut into ribbons

2 cups arugula

1 cup basil leaves, cut into ribbons

1 avocado, medium diced

½ cup toasted pistachios, chopped

¼ cup pomegranate seeds, optional

Directions

- Place shallots in a glass bowl and toss with 1 tablespoon of extra-virgin olive oil and ⅛ teaspoon Himalayan sea salt. Set aside to marinate while you're making the rest of the salad.

- In a blender, purée the garlic, lemon juice, Dijon mustard, and remaining olive oil until smooth. Add ⅛ teaspoon sea salt and pepper.

- In a large bowl, massage kale with the remaining sea salt until the leaves are bright green and tender. Pour in half the dressing and the marinated shallots and toss thoroughly. Taste the kale and add more dressing if desired.

- Fold in the arugula, basil, avocado, and half the pistachios. Top with remaining pistachios and pomegranate seeds. Serve immediately.

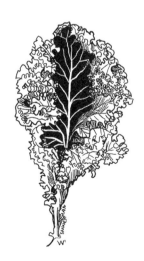

Oodles of Zoodles and Koodles
with Almond Ginger Turmeric Dressing
Serves 4

Ingredients

2 large zucchinis (use 1 yellow summer squash, If possible)

1 medium red bell pepper, seeded and cut into thin strips

1 (7-ounce package) shirataki noodles*

⅓ cup chopped fresh cilantro

½ cup chopped cashews or almonds

1 (2-ounce) package pea shoots

Almond Ginger Turmeric Dressing (see recipe on page 265)

Directions

- Spiralize the zucchini into a large bowl and cut with kitchen scissors so the "zoodles" are about 4 to 5 inches long. If you don't have a spiralizer, peel the zucchini into thin strips with a vegetable peeler.

- Cut the red pepper into thin strips. Add to bowl of spiralized zucchini and toss together. Remove the shirataki noodles from the package and rinse in cold, filtered water. Shake away excess water and toss in with vegetables. Set aside and make *Almond Ginger Turmeric* dressing.

- Pour half the *Dressing* over vegetables and toss to coat thoroughly. Add the cilantro, cashews or almonds, and pea shoots and give the salad another toss. Taste and add more dressing if desired.

HEALTH TIDBIT: *This recipe includes gluten-free, zero-calorie, gelatinous **shirataki** or **konjac noodles**. Made from a water-soluble dietary fiber called glucomannan, shirataki noodles come from the root of the yam-like konjac plant native to Asia. Konjac noodles, which we playfully call **koodles**, may help delay hunger, balance blood sugar, feed friendly bacteria for healthy digestion, and reduce inflammation. Use only the amounts specified in the recipes, because eating more than the recommended serving size may cause bloating, flatulence, or digestive distress.*

Shred-Your-Stress Tahini Ginger Coleslaw

Serves 4

Ingredients

2 cups shredded green cabbage

2 cups shredded purple cabbage

1 cup grated Granny Smith or other tart green apple

1 tablespoon gomasio*

Tahini Ginger Dressing
(see recipe on page 267)

Directions

- Prepare all ingredients and toss together in a bowl. Set aside and make *Tahini Ginger Dressing*. Pour dressing over coleslaw and toss until well distributed.

 CULINARY TERM: Gomasio is a traditional Japanese seasoning blend of toasted sesame seeds, dulse flake or kelp, and sea salt.

To eat is a necessity, but to eat intelligently is an art.[8]

—François de la Rochefoucauld (1613–1680),
noted French author

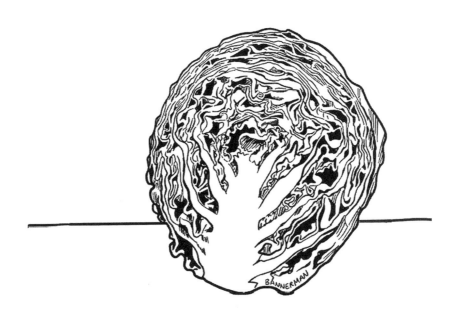

Win-Win Turkey-BLT Salad with Avocado Lime Dressing
Serves 4

Ingredients

4 slices nitrate-free, sugar-free turkey bacon

⅓ oup pcpita seeds

5 cups greens (baby gems or romaine hearts) torn into small pieces

3 ripe tomatoes, sliced into wedges

¼ cup *Avocado Lime Dressing* (see recipe on page 266)

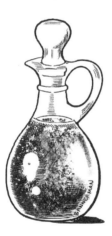

Directions

Preheat the oven to 350°F.

- Place the turkey bacon on a parchment-lined baking sheet and roast in the oven until crispy, about 20 minutes. When bacon is done, use tongs to remove from parchment paper and place on a paper towel to drain. When cooled, break into bite-sized pieces and set aside.

- Toast the pepita seeds in a dry skillet over low heat until they brown lightly and start to pop. Transfer toasted seeds onto a cold plate and allow them to cool. Set aside.

- Make *Avocado Lime Dressing* (see recipe on page 266).

- Pour ¼ cup of the dressing into a salad bowl and gently toss in the lettuce and tomatoes. Taste, and add more dressing if desired. Top with crumbled turkey bacon and toasted pepitas.

SALAD DRESSINGS

On the Bounce Back Diet, you'll learn to make six distinctly different, delicious salad dressings.

 STORAGE POINTERS: *If you have any leftover salad dressing, store it in a Mason jar or another airtight glass container. Label it with the name and date you made it. Creamy dressings will keep for three days in the fridge, while oil-and-vinegar-based dressings will last a week. You can use the remaining salad dressing on salads, roasted vegetables, meat, or fish.*

Garlic Aioli

Ingredients

1 egg yolk

1 garlic clove, minced* to a paste

½ teaspoon Dijon Mustard

½ teaspoon lemon juice

⅛ teaspoon Himalayan sea salt

¼ cup avocado oil

Directions

- Place the egg yolk in a blender and add garlic paste, Dijon mustard, lemon juice, and Himalayan sea salt. Blend until smooth. With the blender on low, add the oil to egg yolk mixture in a steady stream. Continue blending until the aioli is thickened, smooth, and glossy. Taste and adjust seasonings, adding more lemon juice or sea salt as desired.

Almond Ginger Turmeric Dressing

Yield: approximately 1⅓ cups

Ingredients

2-inch piece fresh ginger root or 1 teaspoon ground ginger

1-inch piece fresh turmeric root or ½ teaspoon ground turmeric

3 medium garlic cloves, minced

⅛ teaspoon ground cayenne pepper

1 cup almond butter

¼ cup Bragg Liquid Aminos

2 tablespoons rice vinegar or apple cider vinegar

¼ cup lime juice (about 2 limes)

1 teaspoon toasted sesame oil

3 tablespoons water

⅛ teaspoon freshly cracked pepper

Directions

- Add all the ingredients into a blender and purée until smooth. Taste and adjust seasonings for more heat (cayenne pepper or garlic), tart (lime juice), or savory (Bragg Liquid Aminos).

CULINARY TERM: Mincing *is when you chop food into really tiny pieces.*

Avocado Lime Dressing

Yield: ½ cup

Ingredients

- ½ avocado, pitted
- ¼ teaspoon ground cumin
- ¼ teaspoon oregano
- ¼ teaspoon chili powder, optional
- 1 tablespoon lime juice
- ¼ cup extra-virgin olive oil
- 2 tablespoons water
- ¼ teaspoon Himalayan sea salt

Directions

- Blend all ingredients together in a blender.

Creamy-Better-for-You Ranch Dressing

Yield: Makes 1½ cups

Ingredients

- 1 cup raw, unsalted cashews soaked in filtered water for 2 to 6 hours
- ¾ cup filtered water
- 1½ tablespoon apple cider vinegar
- ½ teaspoon Himalayan sea salt
- 1 small shallot, peeled and ends trimmed
- 1 teaspoon dried Italian seasoning
- 1 garlic clove
- ¼ cup chopped dill
- 2 tablespoons chopped Italian flat-leaf parsley
- ¼ teaspoon freshly cracked black pepper

Directions

- Drain and rinse the cashews and place in a blender with the rest of the ingredients. Purée until smooth. Use this dressing in the Grateful Herb Garden Salad, mixed salad greens, or as a dipping sauce for raw veggies.

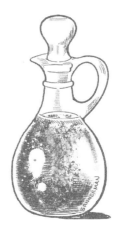

Dazzling Dijon-Shallot Dressing

Yield: Makes about ¾ cup

Ingredients

½ cup champagne or apple cider vinegar

1 small shallot, minced

1 teaspoon Dijon mustard

1 small garlic clove, chopped

¾ cup extra-virgin olive oil

¼ teaspoon Himalayan sea salt

⅛ teaspoon freshly cracked black pepper

Directions

- Add vinegar, shallot, mustard, and garlic to a blender and purée until smooth. Slowly drizzle the olive oil into the blender through the opening in the lid while continuing to blend, until the dressing is smooth. Season with Himalayan sea salt and pepper to taste.

Tahini Ginger Dressing

Yield: about ½ cup

Ingredients

¼ cup tahini

2 tablespoons apple cider vinegar

2 tablespoons Bragg Liquid Aminos

1 teaspoon lemon juice

1 teaspoon, grated fresh ginger

1 scallion, chopped finely

Pinch of sea salt

Directions

- Add all dressing ingredients in a blender and purée until smooth. Use dressing in *Shred-Your-Stress Tahini Ginger Coleslaw* (see page 263).

The food you eat can be either the safest and most powerful form of medicine or the slowest form of poison.[9]

—**Ann Wigmore** (1909–1994), holistic health practitioner, naturopath, raw food advocate, and founder of both the Hippocrates Health Institute in Boston and the Ann Wigmore Natural Health Institute in Puerto Rico

SOUPS

Better-Than-Mom's Chicken Soup

Serves 4

Ingredients

2 tablespoons extra-virgin olive oil or ghee*

1 medium leek, sliced in half lengthwise, cleaned, and cut into thin half moons

1 medium onion, diced

1 fennel bulb, diced

½ teaspoon Himalayan sea salt

4 garlic cloves, chopped finely

¼ teaspoon ground turmeric

4 cups chopped, cooked rotisserie chicken breasts and/or thigh meat

10 cups *Bountiful Bone Broth* (see page 270) or your favorite organic, sugar-free chicken stock

2 large eggs

¼ cup lemon juice, or more to taste

3 cups chopped escarole, chard, collards, or a combination

⅛ teaspoon freshly cracked black pepper

Pinch of Himalayan sea salt or more, to taste

¼ cup chopped fresh dill

Directions

- Heat a large stock pot over medium heat. Add oil and swirl around bottom of pot. Add the leeks, onion, leek, fennel, and Himalayan sea salt. Stir together and cook for about 10 minutes until the onions and leeks soften. Add the garlic and cook for another 2 minutes.

- Sprinkle in turmeric and stir through the vegetables. Cover the pot and allow the vegetables to cook for another 5 minutes until they soften.

- Add in the chicken followed by the stock. Simmer for 15 minutes or until the vegetables are tender.

- Ladle out 1 cup of broth into a small bowl and allow to cool slightly. Whisk the lemon juice and egg yolks into the reserved broth until blended well. Stir the mixture into the soup. Stir gently, lower the heat, and simmer for another 8 minutes.

- Stir in the greens and cook until wilted. Taste, and if desired, add a little more sea salt, pepper, and/or lemon juice. Just before serving, garnish the soup with dill.

CULINARY TERM: Ghee *is a type of clarified butter that's been used in East Asian cooking for thousands of years. When making* **ghee,** *the milk solids and excess water from the butter are removed through simmering and straining. The final result is a lactose-free butter oil that is perfect for cooking foods at high temperatures such as frying or sautéing.*

Creamy Cauliflower Soup
Serves 4

Ingredients

2 tablespoons ghee, extra-virgin olive oil, or avocado oil

1 small onion, diced

2 garlic cloves, diced

¼ teaspoon Himalayan sea salt

½ teaspoon dried thyme

1 large head of cauliflower, chopped (white, orange, or purple)

3–4 cups leftover stock and almond milk mixture from the *Creamy-Dreamy Cauliflower Mash* recipe (see page 280)

⅛ teaspoon ground white pepper

Directions

- Heat a soup or stock pot over medium heat and add the ghee or oil. Add the onions and cook until softened, about 5 minutes. Add the garlic, ¼ teaspoon of Himalayan sea salt, and thyme. Cook for another 1 to 2 minutes until the mixture is very aromatic.

- Add the cauliflower, leftover stock, and almond milk mixture. If the stock doesn't cover the vegetables, add more water. Simmer over medium-low heat until vegetables are fork tender.

- Purée the soup until smooth, using an immersion blender or in batches in a food processor or blender. Add the white pepper and season to taste with a pinch of sea salt and a drizzle of extra-virgin olive oil or ghee, if desired.

Exercise is king. Nutrition is queen.
Put them together, and you've got a kingdom.[10]
—**Jack Lalanne**, *the original celebrity fitness guru*

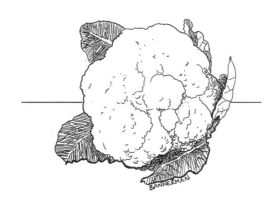

Bountiful Bone Broth

Yield: Makes approximately 5 quarts

Ingredients

4 pounds chicken bones, backs, neck, and wings

1 large onion, chopped

2 celery stalks, chopped

2 bay leaves

1 (4-inch) strip kombu

5 quarts filtered water

1 tablespoon apple cider vinegar

1 teaspoon Himalayan sea salt, optional

Directions

Preheat the oven to 350ºF.

- Place the bones, backs, necks, and wings in a single layer on a large parchment-lined rimmed baking sheet and roast for 1 hour or until the bones are browned.

- Remove the bones from oven and place in a large (12-quart) stock pot. Add the onion, celery, bay leaves, and kombu. Add enough water to cover the bones by two inches. Bring to a boil, then reduce the heat to low so that the broth comes to a simmer.

- Skim off the foam that rises to the top. Once the broth is skimmed, stir in the apple cider vinegar, cover, and simmer for 12 or up to 24 hours.

- Remove the solids with tongs and a slotted spoon. Strain the stock through a sieve lined with cheesecloth into another pot. Season with Himalayan sea salt, if desired.

- Allow the broth to cool for 1 hour before storing in Mason jars. Bone broth can be refrigerated in an airtight jar for one week and kept in the freezer for up to two months. When freezing, be sure to use a food-safe metal or BPA-free container instead of a jar.

 COOKING TIPS: *To make a smaller batch of Bountiful Bone Broth, you can use an Instant Pot®, a slow cooker, or a pressure cooker instead. This recipe makes 5 quarts, so adjust ingredients depending on the size of*

your cooker. A six-quart cooker, for example, makes two quarts of bone broth. Reduce the amount of bones to 1¼ pounds, use half the vegetables, ½ tablespoon of apple cider vinegar, and 2 quarts plus 2 cups of filtered water. If you're cooking the broth for 24 hours, use a slow cooker so you can simmer overnight. Start the slow cooker on high for the first 30 minutes, skim away the foam that rises to the top, then reduce the temperature to low, cover, and cook for 12 to 24 hours. Check the broth periodically and, if needed, add more water to keep the bones covered. If the slow cooker has a timer, you may need to reset it once or twice to continue cooking.

SHOPPING GUIDE: *If you don't have time to cook bone broth from scratch, you can buy it premade. See my blog post at* www.connieb.com/where-to-buy-quality-bone-broth.

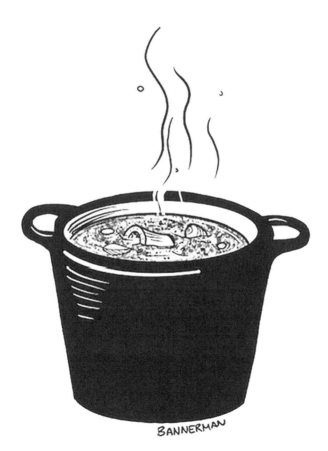

GLUTEN-FREE BREADS

Gluten-free breads will keep for up to seven days in your freezer when you put them in a tightly sealed glass or metal container. To store, first wrap securely in parchment paper.

Refer to your meal plan, the day that you'll eat it, and take a serving of biscuit, focaccia, or muffin out of the freezer. Defrost at room temperature for 1 to 2 hours. For the best flavor, toast lightly or warm up before eating.

Get-Cozy Savory Scallion Almond Biscuits
Makes 6 biscuits

Ingredients

1 tablespoon extra-virgin olive oil

1 cup yellow onion, diced

¾ teaspoon Himalayan sea salt, divided

2 cloves garlic, minced

½ cup ghee

2½ cups almond flour

¼ teaspoon freshly cracked black pepper

1 teaspoon fresh lemon zest*

½ teaspoon baking soda

2 large eggs, whisked slightly

¼ cup unsweetened cashew, almond, or coconut yogurt

2 tablespoons chopped scallions

Directions

Preheat the oven to 325 ºF.

- Line a rimmed baking sheet with parchment paper. Set aside.

- Heat olive oil in a sauté pan or skillet over medium-high heat until oil shimmers. Add the onion and cook until softened. Add ¼ teaspoon Himalayan sea salt and garlic.

- Continue cooking until the onion begins to caramelize, about 8 minutes. Stir frequently to prevent the onion from sticking.

- When onions look soft and golden brown, they're caramelized. At this point, add ghee and stir through the onions until melted. Remove the pan from the heat and set aside.

- In a large bowl, mix the almond flour, remaining ½ teaspoon of sea salt, black pepper, lemon zest, and baking soda. Set aside.

- In another bowl, whisk together the eggs, yogurt, caramelized onions, and ghee. Add to the almond flour mixture and stir until thoroughly mixed. Add the chopped scallions. The dough will be sticky and soft but should hold its shape.

- If the dough is too soft, cover the bowl with parchment paper and chill for 15 minutes in the freezer. When dough is slightly firmer, remove from the freezer and proceed with the recipe.

- Scoop out the dough with a soup spoon to make six round, drop biscuits. Place them two inches apart on prepared baking sheet.

- Bake for 18 to 20 minutes or until the biscuits are golden brown. Allow to cool for 10 minutes and transfer to a baking rack until ready to serve.

 CULINARY TERMS: Lemon zest is finely grated lemon peel, and orange zest comes from a finely grated orange peel.

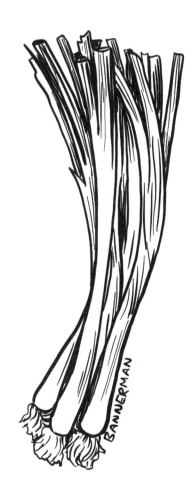

Olive Rosemary Nut-Flax Focaccia

Makes 4 to 6 slices

Ingredients

1 cup walnuts

2 cups almond flour

1½ cups ground flaxseed

1 tablespoon Italian seasoning

1¼ teaspoons Himalayan sea salt, divided

1 teaspoon garlic powder

1 teaspoon baking powder

½ teaspoon baking soda

1 tablespoon apple cider vinegar

½ cup extra-virgin olive oil, divided

2 eggs

10 large green olives, pitted and chopped into small pieces

1 tablespoon dried rosemary

Freshly cracked pepper

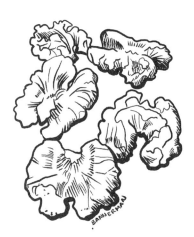

Directions

Preheat the oven to 350°F.

- In a food processor or blender, pulse walnuts to fine crumbs. Add the almond flour, ground flaxseed, Italian seasoning, 1 teaspoon Himalayan sea salt, garlic powder, and baking soda. Pulse until well combined.

- Pour in apple cider vinegar and 6 tablespoons of olive oil, then add the eggs and process until the mixture forms a sticky dough. Turn the dough onto a parchment-lined cutting board and form into a ball. Pat with your palms until dough becomes smoother and less sticky.

- If the dough is too sticky to handle, cover with parchment paper and allow to rest for 10 minutes. The flaxseed will absorb some of the moisture, and the dough will be easier to handle. While the dough is resting, lightly oil a 7" × 11" oven-proof glass baking dish.

- Remove the parchment paper and press the dough into the baking dish. Work quickly and lightly so the dough doesn't stick to your fingers.

- Using your index and middle finger, depress the dough to create dimples across the surface. Drizzle the remaining olive oil across the focaccia and distribute the chopped olives evenly into the dimples. Sprinkle with the rosemary, remaining sea salt, and pepper.

- Bake for 15 to 20 minutes or until a toothpick or skewer inserted into center of the focaccia comes out clean. Allow to cool slightly and slice into triangles or strips.

Zucchini Spice Muffins
Makes 6 muffins

Ingredients

1¼ cups almond flour

¼ teaspoon baking soda

¼ teaspoon Himalayan sea salt

½ teaspoon ground cinnamon

¼ teaspoon vanilla powder or vanilla extract

2 tablespoons coconut oil, melted, or avocado oil

2 tablespoons almond butter or other nut butter

2 eggs

¼ cup grated zucchini

Directions

Preheat the oven to 375 °F.

- Line a 6-cup muffin tin or a baking pan with 6 muffin cups.

- In a medium bowl, mix the almond flour, baking soda, Himalayan sea salt, cinnamon, and vanilla powder together and set aside.

- In a large bowl, stir together the oil and almond butter until smooth. Add the eggs one at a time, stirring well after each addition. Add the almond flour mixture and stir until well combined. Fold in the grated zucchini.

- Distribute the batter evenly into the paper cups and bake for 15 to 20 minutes or until a toothpick inserted in center of a muffin comes out clean.

Forget calories. Focus on quality.
Let your body do the rest.[11]

—**David Ludwig, MD**, endocrinologist, researcher
and author of *Always Hungry?*

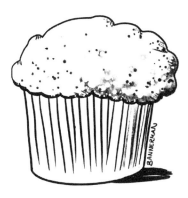

SPREADS

In-a-Hurry Sunflower Avocado Tuna Spread
Yield: about 1¾ cups

Ingredients

1 (5-ounce) can wild Albacore tuna, drained

1 tablespoon Primal Mayo or *Garlic Aioli* (see recipe on page 265)

1 teaspoon Dijon mustard

½ teaspoon lemon juice

¼ cup diced celery

¼ cup diced red bell pepper

1 tablespoon toasted sunflower seeds

2 teaspoons hemp seeds

1 small avocado, diced

¼ teaspoon Himalayan sea salt

⅛ teaspoon freshly cracked pepper

Directions

- Place the tuna in a medium bowl and break up the pieces with a fork. Stir in the mayo, mustard, and lemon juice. Gently fold in the celery, red pepper, sunflower seeds, hemp seeds, and avocado. Season with Himalayan sea salt and pepper.

- Serve immediately or store in an airtight container for up to two days in the refrigerator.

Oh-So-Good Olive Walnut Tapenade
Yield: ½ cup

Ingredients

1 cup of your favorite olives, black, green, or mixed, pits removed

½ tablespoon capers, drained

¼ cup walnuts, toasted and chopped

1 small garlic clove, chopped

1 tablespoon chopped Italian flat-leaf parsley

1 tablespoon chopped fresh dill

1 tablespoon chopped fresh tarragon, optional

2 tablespoons extra-virgin olive oil

Juice and zest of 1 lemon

Directions

- Place the olives, capers, walnuts, garlic clove, parsley, dill, tarragon (if using), and olive oil in a food processor and pulse until coarse and chunky.

- You also can chop the ingredients by hand. Transfer to a bowl and stir in lemon zest and juice to taste.

Zesty Lemon Pepper Zucchini Tahini Spread

Makes approximately 1 cup

Ingredients

1 medium zucchini

Avocado oil

Pinch of Himalayan sea salt

Pinch of freshly cracked black pepper

2 tablespoons pistachios

1 large garlic clove

2 tablespoons tahini

2 tablespoons extra-virgin olive oil

1½ tablespoons lemon juice

Himalayan sea salt, to taste

Freshly cracked black pepper, to taste

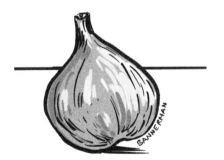

Directions

Preheat the oven to 375ºF.

- Line a rimmed baking sheet with parchment paper.

- Slice the zucchini in half lengthwise. Brush each side generously with avocado oil and sprinkle with a pinch each of sea salt and pepper. Place on prepared baking sheet. Roast for 20 minutes until soft and lightly browned. Remove the zucchini from oven and allow to cool slightly.

- While the zucchini is cooling, grind pistachios into a fine crumb. If you don't have a spice grinder, use a food processor or blender and pulse several times to a nut meal consistency. You also can grind the nuts by hand using a mortar and pestle.

- Once the zucchini has cooled, roughly chop and add the pieces to a food processor or blender along with the garlic, tahini, olive oil, and lemon juice.

- Process until smooth and creamy. Taste and adjust seasoning with more lemon juice, sea salt, and pepper, if desired.

If it came from a plant, eat it;
if it was made in a plant, don't.[12]

—Michael Pollan, bestselling author of
In Defense of Food: An Eater's Manifesto

VEGETABLES

Cauliflower Couscous with Basil Arugula Pesto

Serves 4

Ingredients

Basil Arugula Pesto

1 cup arugula

¾ cup basil leaves

¼ cup walnuts

2 cloves garlic

Zest and juice of 1 lemon

½ cup extra-virgin olive oil

¼ teaspoon Himalayan sea salt

⅛ teaspoon freshly cracked black pepper

Cauliflower Couscous

2 medium heads cauliflower (white, orange, or purple)

2 tablespoons extra-virgin olive oil

1 large red onion, diced

¼ teaspoon Himalayan sea salt

¼ cup fresh basil leaves

Directions

Make the pesto:

- Add the arugula, basil, walnuts, garlic, lemon zest, lemon juice, and olive oil to a blender. Purée until smooth. Season to taste with Himalayan sea salt and pepper. Set aside.

Make the couscous:

- Cut the cauliflower into florets and put into a food processor. Pulse the cauliflower into a grain-like consistency or use a chef's knife to cut the cauliflower into small, crumbly pieces.

- Heat a large sauté pan and add the olive oil, followed by red onion. Cook until the onion is softened, about 5 minutes. Add the cauliflower and sea salt. Cook until softened, about 15 minutes. Pour in half the pesto and stir to coat the cauliflower. Cook for another 10 minutes.

- Add more pesto to your taste. Season with salt and pepper. Transfer to a platter, and garnish with freshly torn basil.

Confetti Brussels Sprouts with Leeks and Turkey-Bacon

Serves 4

Ingredients

1 pound of Brussels sprouts, shredded

1 leek, well washed and sliced thinly

5 slices turkey bacon, diced

¼ cup extra-virgin olive oil

1 tablespoon apple cider vinegar

1 teaspoon Dijon mustard

½ teaspoon Himalayan sea salt

¼ teaspoon freshly cracked black pepper

Directions

Preheat the oven 375ºF.

- Line a rimmed baking sheet with parchment paper.

- Place shredded Brussel sprouts, sliced leek, and turkey bacon in a large bowl and stir to combine.

- In a small bowl, whisk together the olive oil, apple cider vinegar, mustard, Himalayan sea salt, and pepper. Toss the dressing with the vegetables until they're evenly coated.

- Transfer to the prepared baking sheet, and roast for 25 minutes or until the vegetables are lightly browned.

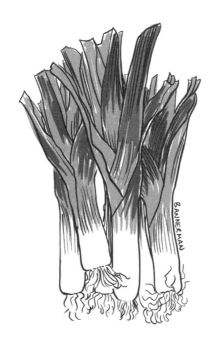

Creamy-Dreamy Cauliflower Mash

Serves 6

Ingredients

1 whole garlic head

2 tablespoons extra-virgin olive oil

10 cups of white cauliflower florets (about 2 small heads or 1 large head of white cauliflower)

1 quart unsweetened almond or coconut milk

3 cups Bountiful Bone Broth or vegetable stock

2 bay leaves

1 teaspoon Himalayan sea salt

1 teaspoon thyme

2 tablespoons ghee or extra-virgin olive oil

Freshly cracked black pepper, to taste

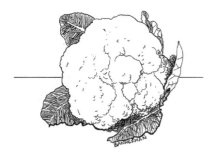

Directions

Preheat the oven to 350°F.

- Tear off a piece of foil big enough to enclose the head of garlic. Lay a piece of parchment paper of the same size on top of it.

- Make a shallow cut across the stem end of the garlic head, and drizzle olive oil over the exposed cloves. Wrap the garlic in the parchment and foil, and roast in the oven for 1 hour or until cloves are buttery soft.

- Allow the garlic to cool before handling. Unwrap the garlic and squeeze out softened cloves into a bowl. Mash garlic with a fork to form a paste.

- While garlic is roasting, add the cauliflower florets to a large pot, along with the almond or coconut milk, bone broth or vegetable stock, bay leaves, olive oil, and Himalayan sea salt.

- Bring the mixture to a boil. Reduce the heat to low and simmer for 15 to 20 minutes or until the cauliflower is fork tender. Drain the cauliflower, reserving the liquid for Creamy Cauliflower Soup (see recipe on page 269).

- Place the cauliflower in a large bowl and add the thyme, ghee or olive oil, and garlic clove paste. Using an immersion blender, purée until smooth. Alternatively, you can use a potato masher. Season with a pinch or more sea salt and pepper to taste.

Feels-Like-I'm-Cheating Creamed Greens
Serves 6

Ingredients

5 bunches of kale, chard, collards, or a combination of all three, stemmed

1 tablespoon avocado oil

1 small onion, diced

¼ teaspoon Himalayan sea salt

1 garlic clove, minced

Freshly cracked pepper, to taste

Silky Pecan Cream Sauce (see recipe on page 282)

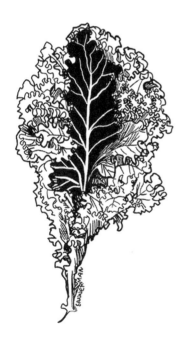

Directions

- Wash and pat dry greens and chop into bite-sized pieces. Set aside.

- Heat a large sauté pan over medium heat and add the avocado oil. Swirl the oil around in the pan. Add the onions and cook for 3 to 5 minutes until softened and translucent. Sprinkle in the Himalayan sea salt. Reduce the heat to low and cook the onions for 10 more minutes or until golden brown and very soft.

- Remove 2 tablespoons of the cooked onions and set aside in a small bowl for making *Silky Pecan Cream Sauce*. (see recipe on page 282).

- Add the garlic to remaining onions and cook for another minute until aromatic.

- Add the chopped greens and cook until the greens start to wilt. Continue cooking for another 5 minutes.

- Pour in the *Silky Pecan Cream Sauce*. Cook on low heat for another 10 minutes. Add sea salt and more pepper to taste. Serve immediately.

Silky Pecan Cream Sauce

Ingredients

2 tablespoons cooked onions

1 cup pecans, soaked for 2 hours, drained and rinsed

1½ cups vegetable stock

½ teaspoon garlic powder

½ teaspoon Himalayan sea salt

1 tablespoon extra-virgin olive oil

Pinch of nutmeg

Directions

- Put the cooked onions into a blender.

- Add pecans, stock, garlic powder, Himalayan sea salt, olive oil, and nutmeg.

- Blend until smooth and creamy.

Kale Chip Krispies

Serves 2

Ingredients

2 tablespoons apple cider vinegar

¼ cup extra-virgin olive oil

2 teaspoons Dijon mustard

1 bunch kale (lacinato or dinosaur), stem removed, cut into 3-inch pieces

1 bunch of curly kale, stems removed

½ teaspoon of Himalayan sea salt

¼ teaspoon freshly cracked black pepper

Directions

Preheat the oven to 350°F.

- Line a rimmed baking sheet with parchment paper.

- Whisk the vinegar, oil, and mustard in a large bowl. Add all the kale and toss to coat lightly. Sprinkle in sea salt and pepper.

- Place the kale in a single layer on the prepared baking sheets. Bake for 10 to 15 minutes or until kale leaves are crisp. Remove from oven and allow to cool.

 STORAGE POINTERS: *Store the Kale Chip Krispies in an airtight container. They will keep for up to three days. If they soften, preheat the oven to 250°F and place on a baking sheet for 5 to 8 minutes or until crispy.*

Oven Cauli "Fries"
Serves 4

Ingredients

1 large head of white cauliflower, broken up into florets

3 tablespoons avocado or extra-virgin olive oil

1 teaspoon ground cumin

½ teaspoon ground paprika

¼ teaspoon Himalayan sea salt

¼ teaspoon coriander

⅛ teaspoon ground white pepper

Directions

Preheat the oven to 400°F.

- Line a rimmed baking sheet with parchment paper.

- Place the cauliflower florets in a large bowl. Add the oil and toss to coat the cauliflower.

- In a small bowl, mix the cumin, paprika, Himalayan sea salt, coriander, and white pepper. Sprinkle over the cauliflower and toss to coat. Arrange cauliflower in a single layer on the prepared baking sheet.

- Bake for 20 minutes or until the cauliflower is lightly browned and crisp on the outside and soft on the inside. The cauliflower is done when a fork pierces the thickest piece with ease. If the cauliflower is still firm, roast in the oven for another 8 to 10 minutes. Serve immediately.

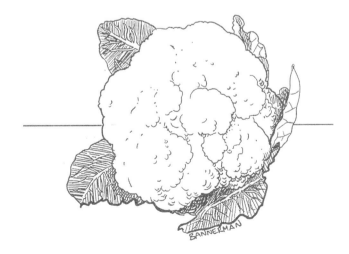

Spaghetti Squash Noodles
Serves 4

Ingredients

1 medium spaghetti squash (about 3 pounds)

1 tablespoon melted avocado oil

Pinch of Himalayan sea salt

1 tablespoon extra-virgin olive oil

Directions

Preheat the oven to 350°F.

- Line a rimmed baking sheet with parchment paper.

- Cut the spaghetti squash in half crosswise and scoop out the seeds.

- Brush the cut sides with avocado oil and place cut side down on the prepared baking sheet. Bake for 25 minutes or until squash is tender when pricked with a knife. Remove the squash from the oven and cool for 10 minutes.

- Using a fork, scrape the strands of spaghetti squash out of the skin and place into a bowl.

- Add a pinch of Himalayan sea salt and 1 tablespoon of the olive oil. Toss lightly and set aside until ready to use.

 COOKING TIP: *You can gently reheat spaghetti squash in a skillet with your sauce of choice.*

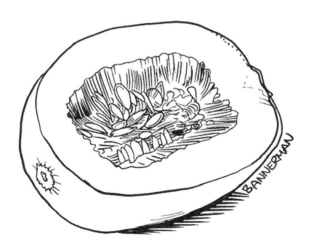

Stir-Fried Broccolini and Bok Choy with Crispy Shiitake Mushrooms

Serves 4

Ingredients

1 pound shiitake mushrooms, stems removed

¼ cup avocado oil, divided

Himalayan sea salt and pepper, to taste

2 teaspoons Bragg Liquid Aminos

1 tablespoon miso paste

1 tablespoon rice vinegar

1 tablespoon toasted sesame oil

¼ teaspoon chili flakes, optional

1 tablespoon avocado oil

3 garlic cloves, sliced thinly

1-inch piece fresh ginger, minced

2 shallots, sliced

3 bunches baby bok choy greens, chopped, stems and greens in separate piles

3 bunches broccolini or broccoli, stems removed, and florets cut into small pieces

1 tablespoon gomasio or toasted sesame seeds

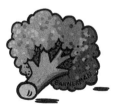

Directions

Preheat the oven to 350°F.

- Line a rimmed baking sheet with parchment paper.

- Slice the shiitake mushrooms thinly and spread out evenly onto the prepared baking sheet. Brush each slice lightly with avocado oil and sprinkle with Himalayan sea salt and pepper. Roast for 20 minutes until mushrooms start to look crispy. Turn off the oven and leave the mushrooms to dry out, about 20 more minutes.

- In a small bowl, combine the Bragg Liquid Aminos, miso, vinegar, sesame oil, and chili flakes if desired. Add 1 to 2 tablespoons of water if needed to bring sauce together into a smooth, pourable paste.

- Heat a pan or wok over high heat. Sprinkle a few drops of water onto the surface. If the water quickly forms a bead and sizzles away, the pan is ready to use. Add the remaining avocado oil and swirl around evenly to coat the bottom of the pan. Quickly add the garlic and ginger and stir-fry until aromatic. This will take about 30 seconds.

- Add the shallots and cook for another minute, then add the bok choy stems and broccolini florets. Stir-fry for another minute.

- Add the bok choy leaves and cook until greens just start to wilt and turn bright green, about 2 to 3 minutes more. Turn off the heat.

- Add the miso mixture to vegetables and stir well to coat.

- Top with crispy shiitake mushrooms and gomasio or toasted sesame seeds. Serve immediately.

Thyme-Scented Green Beans with Chopped Almonds
Serves 4

Ingredients

2 tablespoons avocado oil

2 medium shallots, minced (about 1/3 cup)

¼ teaspoon Himalayan sea salt

1 teaspoon thyme leaves

4 cups sliced green beans (slice longer ones into thirds)

2 tablespoons apple cider vinegar

½ cup chopped dry roasted almonds

Directions

- Heat a sauté pan or wok over medium low heat. Add 1 tablespoon of avocado oil. Swirl the oil around in the bottom of the pan. Add the shallots and cook for about 4 minutes. Add the sea salt and thyme and continue cooking until shallots are translucent.

- Add the green beans and increase the heat to medium. Cook for 2 to 3 minutes, stirring frequently. Stir in the apple cider vinegar. Fold in the chopped almonds.

- Reduce the heat to low and cook until the green beans are tender crisp. This should take another 8 minutes or so. Add another pinch or two of sea salt and freshly cracked pepper. Serve immediately.

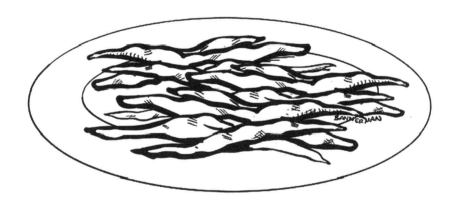

BREAKFAST AND LUNCH

As-You-Like-It Frittata

Serves 4 to 6

Ingredients

1 medium onion, sauté slice*

2 tablespoons avocado oil, divided

1¼ teaspoons Himalayan sea salt

½ teaspoon garlic powder

4 cups stemmed and chopped escarole, kale, or chard leaves, or a combination of all three

8 eggs

½ cup unsweetened coconut, almond, or cashew milk

1 cup leftover salmon or chicken, optional

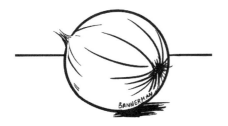

Directions

Preheat the oven to 350°F.

- Heat an eight-inch sauté pan or cast-iron skillet and add the avocado oil.

- Add the onion and cook for 5 minutes, stirring frequently. Sprinkle in the sea salt and garlic powder. Cook for another 8 minutes until onions become very soft.

- Add the chopped greens and cook for another 3 to 5 minutes. Remove the pan from heat and set aside.

- In a large bowl, whisk the eggs with nut milk and fold in the cooked vegetables. If you're using salmon or chicken, add to the egg mixture.

- Wipe down the pan and heat it over medium heat with the remaining oil. Make sure the fat coats the bottom of pan. Turn off the heat and pour the egg mixture into the hot pan. Gently move the eggs and vegetable mixture around to distribute evenly.

- Place the pan in the preheated oven and bake for 50 minutes or until it sets. The eggs should be slightly wet in the middle and not slosh in the pan. Remove the frittata from the oven when ready. Let it continue to cook in the pan at room temperature. To serve, slice into wedges and enjoy one slice on its own or with a tossed green salad.

 CULINARY TERM: *To cut an onion in **sauté slice**, cut it in half from the stem end to the root end. Remove skin and cut into long slices, along the pinstripe of the onion.*

Sassy-Saucy Poached Eggs with Rainbow Chard
Serves 4

Ingredients

2 tablespoons extra-virgin olive oil

1 bunch rainbow chard, leaves removed from stems and chopped, stems diced

1 small onion, finely chopped

2 garlic cloves, coarsely chopped

Pinch of Himalayan salt

1 jalapeño, seeded and finely chopped, optional

1 teaspoon ground paprika

½ teaspoon ground cumin

1 (14-ounce) can diced organic tomatoes

Pinch of freshly cracked black pepper

4 large eggs

1 cup chopped cilantro or parsley

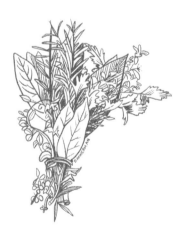

Directions

Preheat the oven to 425°F.

- Heat the oil in a 10-inch-sized ovenproof skillet over medium-high heat. Add the chard stems, onion, garlic, a pinch of Himalayan sea salt, and jalapeños if desired. Cook, stirring occasionally, until onion is soft, about 8 minutes.

- Add the paprika and cumin and cook for 2 minutes longer.

- Add tomatoes and their juices. Bring to a gentle boil, reduce the heat to medium-low, and simmer, stirring occasionally, until sauce thickens slightly, about 15 minutes. Season to taste with sea salt and pepper.

- Gently stir the chard leaves through sauce.

- Crack the eggs one at a time into a small, heat-proof bowl (a ramekin or custard cup works well). Carefully tip the ramekin or bowl into the pan so each egg slides gently into the sauce. Space the eggs evenly so they're not touching.

- Place a lid over the skillet and cook until the egg whites are opaque and yolks are cooked as you like. For runny yolks, cook 5 to 8 minutes, or for firmer yolks, cook for 10 to 15 minutes. To serve, sprinkle with cilantro or parsley and enjoy.

Sumptuous Seasonal Scrambled Eggs

Serves 1

Ingredients

1 tablespoon avocado oil or ghee

3 large eggs, beaten well with a fork

2 scallions, white and green parts, sliced

1 small garlic clove, minced

¼ teaspoon Himalayan sea salt, and a pinch more, to taste

Freshly cracked black pepper, to taste

Delicious Seasonal Additions, if desired (see page 290)

Directions

- Heat a ceramic-lined nonstick skillet or frying pan over medium heat. Add the oil or ghee and swirl around to coat the bottom of the pan. Add the scallions and cook until softened. Add the Himalayan sea salt and garlic and continue to cook for 1 minute, moving vegetables frequently with a heat-proof spatula so the garlic doesn't burn.

- Pour in the eggs and gently move the mixture around the pan with the spatula until the scramble is your desired consistency. Taste and adjust seasonings with a pinch of sea salt and pepper. If desired, make the scramble with *Delicious Seasonal Additions* below.

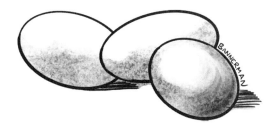

Delicious Seasonal Additions

Springtime Veggie Renewal

Ingredients

½ cup trimmed and sliced green beans or asparagus

Chopped fresh dill, Italian flat-leaf parsley, chervil, or cilantro

¼ teaspoon lemon zest

1 teaspoon ghee, softened

Himalayan sea salt to taste, optional

Directions

- Steam green beans or asparagus until tender and bright green and toss with ghee, fresh herbs, lemon zest, and Himalayan sea salt to taste. Serve on top of scrambled eggs.

Summertime Tomato Basil Scramble

Ingredients

⅓ cup cherry tomatoes, sliced

2 tablespoons chopped, fresh basil leaves

Directions

- Add cherry tomatoes in the Sumptuous *Seasonal Scrambled Eggs,* recipe on page 289, and cook for 2 minutes before adding the beaten egg mixture. Top with basil.

Fall Brussels, Turkey-Bacon 'n Egg Scramble

Ingredients

1 tablespoon extra-virgin olive oil

4 Brussels sprouts, thinly sliced

¼ teaspoon Himalayan sea salt

¼ teaspoon lemon juice

2 slices turkey bacon, cooked and crumbled

Directions

- Heat a skillet over medium heat and add the oil. Add the Brussels sprouts and Himalayan sea salt and cook until softened, about 10 minutes. Stir in lemon juice and fold in cooked and crumbled turkey bacon.
- Add mixture to the scallions and garlic in the Sumptuous Seasonal Scrambled Eggs (recipe on page 289).

Winter Roasted Curried Cauliflower Scramble

Ingredients

2 teaspoons coconut oil, melted

¼ teaspoon curry powder

⅛ teaspoon garlic powder

⅛ teaspoon ground cumin

¼ teaspoon Himalayan sea salt

1½ cups cauliflower florets, white, orange, or purple

1 tablespoon finely chopped cilantro

Directions

Preheat the oven to 375°F.

- Line a rimmed baking sheet with parchment paper.

- Add the melted coconut oil to a medium bowl and whisk in the spices and Himalayan sea salt. Toss the cauliflower with the coconut oil and spice mixture. Spread in a single layer on the prepared baking sheet.

- Roast for 20 minutes, or until cauliflower is lightly browned and tender when pricked with a fork. Fold the roasted cauliflower into the cooked Sumptuous Seasonal Scrambled Eggs and top with cilantro.

A healthy diet is a solution to many of our health-care problems. It's the most important solution.[13]

—**John Mackey**, entrepreneur, cofounder, and former CEO of Whole Foods Market

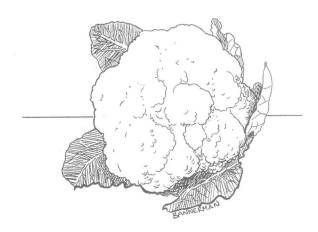

DINNER

Crazy-Good Crab Cakes

Serves 4

Ingredients

½ **pound crab meat**

2 tablespoons red bell pepper, diced

1 tablespoon *Garlic Aioli*
(see recipe on page 265)

1 tablespoon minced scallion, white and green parts

¼ **tablespoon minced Italian flat-leaf parsley**

2 tablespoons almond flour

1 egg white (reserve yolk for Garlic Aioli, recipe on page 265)

1 tablespoon avocado oil

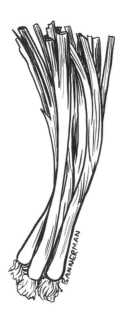

Directions

- Line a rimmed baking sheet or sheet pan with parchment paper.

- Gently stir together the crab, red bell pepper, scallion, parsley, Garlic Aioli, almond flour, and egg white until mixed well. Place six rounded scoops on the prepared sheet pan and press each mound down gently into a circular shape that's about 1-inch thick and 3-inches in diameter. Cover the crab cakes with parchment paper and chill in the refrigerator for 15 to 30 minutes.

- Heat the flat side of a griddle, cast iron pan, or ceramic-lined nonstick pan over medium high heat. Brush the griddle with oil, and cook the crab cakes on each side until evenly browned and internal temperature reads 165°F with a meat thermometer.

- Transfer the crab cakes to an oven-proof platter or plate and cover lightly with foil. Keep crab cakes in a warm oven until ready to serve.

Crispy Provençal Chicken Thighs

Serves 4

Ingredients

1½ teaspoons Himalayan sea salt

½ teaspoon freshly cracked black pepper

1 tablespoon dried oregano

1 tablespoon dried thyme

2 tablespoons dried rosemary

3 cloves garlic, smashed and minced

¼ cup extra-virgin olive oil, divided

2 fennel bulbs, tops and outer layers removed, cored, and sliced crosswise

4 shallots, chopped

2 red bell peppers, stemmed, seeded, and chopped

1 cup cherry tomatoes, sliced in half

½ cup pitted green olives

2 tablespoons lemon juice

1¼ cups *Bountiful Bone Broth* (see recipe on page 270) **or good quality, store-bought bone broth or chicken stock**

6 skin-on, bone-in chicken thighs

Directions

Preheat the oven to 375°F.

- In a small bowl mix together the sea salt, pepper, oregano, thyme, rosemary, and garlic.

- In a large bowl, whisk 2 tablespoons olive oil with half the garlic and herb mixture. Add the fennel, shallots, red pepper, tomatoes, and olives and toss to coat thoroughly.

- Layer the seasoned vegetables into a large roasting pan. Stir together the lemon juice with the broth and pour over the vegetables.

- In the same large bowl, whisk together the remaining olive oil and garlic and herb mixture. Add chicken thighs and toss gently to coat them. Nestle the chicken thighs on top of the vegetables. Don't allow the broth to cover the skin.

- Roast for 45 minutes to one hour, or until the chicken skin looks crispy and a meat thermometer reads 165°F when inserted in the thickest portion of chicken thighs, and juices run clear.

Golden Power Skirt Steak

Serves 4

Ingredients

1 medium onion, chopped (about 1 cup)

2 garlic cloves

1-inch piece fresh ginger root or 1 teaspoon ground ginger

1-inch piece fresh turmeric root or ½ teaspoon ground turmeric

¼ cup avocado oil

¼ cup Bragg Liquid Aminos

¼ teaspoon Himalayan sea salt

¼ teaspoon freshly cracked black pepper

1¼ pounds skirt or flank steak

Directions

- Place the onion, garlic, ginger, turmeric, avocado oil, Bragg Liquid Aminos, sea salt, and pepper in a blender and purée until smooth.

- Place the skirt steak in an oven-proof glass baking dish and pour the marinade over it, coating it well on both sides. Cover the dish tightly with a lid and allow the steak to marinate for 4 hours or overnight.

- When ready to cook, remove the steak from the marinade and shake off the excess liquid. Pat dry with paper towels.

- Place in a broiler pan and broil for 4 minutes on each side until medium rare. You can also cook these steaks on your outdoor grill for about the same amount of time.

- Remove the steaks from the heat and allow to rest for a few minutes. Cut across the grain into 1-inch-wide strips.

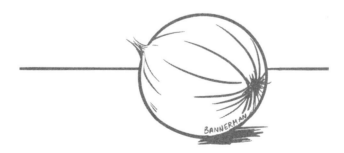

Healing Slow Roasted Chicken with Lemons, Olives, and Capers

Serves 4

Ingredients

Marinade:

½ cup extra-virgin olive oil

4 bay leaves

6 garlic cloves, minced

½ cup capers with juice

1 cup green olives, pitted

½ cup lemon juice

¼ cup Italian seasoning blend

1¼ teaspoons Himalayan sea salt

½ teaspoon pepper

2 lemons, thinly sliced and seeds removed

4 bone-in, skin-on chicken thighs

2 bone-in, skin-on chicken breasts

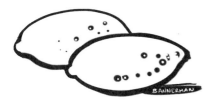

Directions

The day before you roast the chicken, make the marinade:

- Combine the olive oil, bay leaves, garlic, capers, olives, lemon juice, Italian seasonings, Himalayan sea salt, pepper, and lemon slices in a glass container large enough to hold the chicken pieces. Add the chicken and coat well with marinade. Cover and marinate overnight in the refrigerator.

The next day:

- Take the chicken out of the fridge and allow it to sit at room temperature for 1 hour.

Preheat the oven to 350°F.

- Arrange the chicken in a large oven-proof baking dish. Top each piece of chicken with marinated lemon slices and distribute remaining marinade evenly around chicken.

- Roast the chicken for 1 hour or until a meat thermometer reads 165°F, when inserted in the thickest portion of a piece of chicken breast, and juices run clear. Check the temperature of the thighs since they sometimes take slightly longer to cook. If the thighs need to cook longer, remove the breasts and keep them warm so they don't overcook.

Herby Turkey Meatballs with Garlicky Basil Cream Sauce

Yield: 8 golf ball-sized meatballs
Serving size: 4 meatballs

Ingredients

2 tablespoons extra-virgin olive oil

1 medium onion, finely diced (about 2 cups)

6 cloves garlic, minced

¼ teaspoon Himalayan sea salt

¼ teaspoon ground white pepper

⅛ teaspoon freshly cracked black pepper

1 teaspoon Italian seasoning

1 tablespoon Za'atar,* optional

1 tablespoon Dijon mustard

2 pounds ground turkey thigh

¼ cup Italian flat-leaf parsley

½ cup almond flour

1 large egg

¼ cup avocado oil, divided

Garlicky Basil Cream Sauce
(see recipe on page 298)

Directions

- Heat a large sauté pan over medium heat with olive oil. Add the onions and cook while stirring frequently for about 2 to 5 minutes until they become soft and translucent. Add the garlic, sea salt, white pepper, black pepper, Italian seasoning, and Za'atar.

- Cook while stirring constantly for 2 minutes until the spices and onions become aromatic. Stir in the mustard and remove the pan from the heat.

- Place the ground turkey in a large bowl and add the cooked onion mixture. Stir well with a wooden spoon or incorporate mixture thoroughly with your hands.

- Add the parsley and almond flour and mix evenly. Whip the egg in a small bowl and add to the meatball mixture. Combine thoroughly. Test seasoning by forming about ½ tablespoon of the ground turkey mixture into a miniburger.

- Heat a small pan over medium heat, lightly coat the pan with avocado oil, and cook the burger until it no longer looks pink. Taste and decide if you want to add more sea salt and pepper. Once you're satisfied with the flavor, make your meatballs.

- Line a baking sheet tray with parchment paper. Grab a slightly larger-than-a-golf-ball-size of meat mixture and roll into a ball. Don't pack it too tightly, but make sure meatball is formed well enough to stay together.

- Once meatballs are rolled and ready, cover sheet pan with parchment paper and chill for at least 30 minutes.

Preheat the oven to 350°F.

- Heat a large sauté pan and add 2 tablespoons of avocado oil. Brown the meatballs on all sides. Don't cook them all the way through. Continue until all meatballs are browned, adding remaining avocado oil, if needed, to keep the pan from becoming too dry.

- As the meatballs become browned, place them on a parchment-lined baking sheet. Place the meatballs in the preheated oven and bake for 15 to 20 minutes or until meat thermometer inserted in the middle of meatball reads 165°F.

- Serve meatballs on top of *Spaghetti Squash Noodles* with *Garlicky Basil Cream Sauce*.

 CULINARY TERM: Za'atar is a popular Middle Eastern spice blend that typically includes a combination of savory dried herbs such as oregano, thyme, or marjoram, along with toasted earthy spices like cumin and coriander, combined with sesame seeds, salt, and sumac. It can enliven many different foods such as cucumbers, hard-boiled eggs, chickpeas, chicken, or turkey.

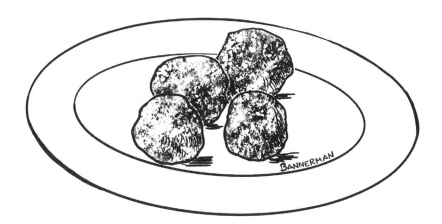

Garlicky Basil Cream Sauce

Makes about 3½ cups

Ingredients

1 cup cashews,* soaked in filtered water for 2 to 6 hours

2 cups tightly packed basil leaves

1 cup vegetable stock

¼ cup extra-virgin olive oil

3 garlic cloves

½ teaspoon Dijon mustard

½ teaspoon lemon juice, or more, to taste

½ teaspoon Himalayan sea salt

Freshly cracked black pepper, to taste

Directions

- Drain and rinse the cashews and add to a blender along with basil, vegetable stock, olive oil, garlic cloves, mustard, lemon juice, sea salt, and pepper. Purée until smooth, Taste and add a touch more olive oil, lemon juice, or sea salt to taste.

- Gently heat sauce in a saucepan before ladling onto Herby Turkey Meatballs.

 COOKING TIP: *Soaking cashews in water for 2 to 6 hours softens them so that they easily blend to a smooth consistency. Rinse the cashews well after soaking. If you're short on time, simmer the nuts for ten minutes, drain, and proceed with the recipe.*

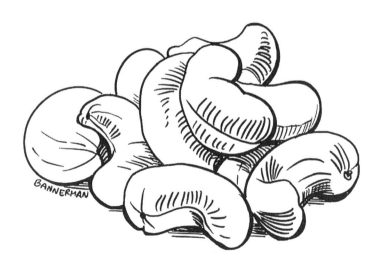

Pistachio Crusted Halibut
Serves 4

Ingredients

2 cups pistachios

4 halibut fillets, about 4 ounces each

Smoked Paprika Sauce

2 tablespoons Primal Kitchen Mayo or *Garlic Aioli* (see recipe on page 265)

½ teaspoon smoked paprika

½ teaspoon garlic powder

1 teaspoon lemon juice

¼ teaspoon Himalayan sea salt

⅛ teaspoon freshly cracked black pepper 1 lemon, thinly sliced, seeds removed

Directions

Preheat the oven 350°F.

- Line a rimmed baking sheet with parchment paper.

- Using a blender or food processor, pulse the pistachios into coarse crumbs. Place them into a small bowl and set aside.

- In another small bowl, stir the Primal Kitchen Mayo or *Garlic Aioli*, smoked paprika, garlic powder, lemon juice, sea salt, and black pepper together until smooth.

- Place the halibut fillets on the prepared baking sheet. Brush both sides with Smoked Paprika Sauce.

- Carefully press the pistachio crumbs evenly onto both sides of fish. Top with thinly sliced lemons. Bake for 8 to 10 minutes or until the fish flakes easily with a fork.

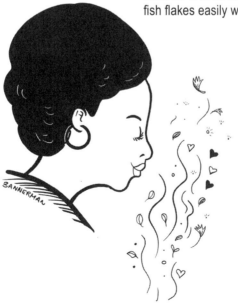

Moroccan Cottage Pie
Serves 6

Ingredients

Celery Root Mash

1 whole garlic head

1 tablespoon ghee or extra-virgin olive oil

1 large celery root, peeled and chopped (about 4 cups)

1½ teaspoon Himalayan sea salt, divided

1 tablespoon coconut oil

½ cup full-fat, unsweetened coconut milk

¼ teaspoon garam masala*

Pinch cayenne

Filling

1 tablespoon ghee or extra-virgin olive oil

1 medium onion, small diced (about 1 cup)

2 celery stalks, small diced (about ½ cup)

2 garlic cloves, minced

1 teaspoon garam masala

½ teaspoon ground cinnamon

¼ teaspoon whole fennel seeds

¼ teaspoon ground turmeric

1 teaspoon Himalayan sea salt

½ teaspoon freshly cracked black pepper

½ pound button mushrooms, chopped

½ pound ground turkey thigh meat

½ pound ground bison or beef

1 tablespoon almond flour

2 cups *Bountiful Bone Broth* (see recipe on page 270) **or good quality, store-bought bone broth or chicken stock**

Directions

Preheat the oven to 350°F.

- Tear off a piece of foil big enough to enclose the head of garlic. Lay a piece of parchment paper of the same size on top of the foil.

- Make a shallow cut across the stem end of the garlic head, and drizzle olive oil over the exposed cloves. Wrap the garlic in the parchment and foil, and roast in the oven for one hour or until cloves are buttery soft.

- Allow the garlic to cool before handling. When cooled, unwrap the garlic and squeeze out the softened cloves into a bowl. Mash with a fork to form a paste. Set aside.

- Place the peeled and chopped celery root in a pot, cover with water and bring to a boil. When water is boiling, add 1 teaspoon of sea salt. Cook until the celery root is fork tender. Drain and set aside.

- In a large sauté pan, heat 1 tablespoon of ghee or olive oil, and cook the onions and celery while stirring frequently until softened, about 2 to 4 minutes.

- Add the garlic, garam masala, cinnamon, fennel seeds, turmeric, sea salt, and pepper. Stir through vegetables to coat evenly. Cook while stirring constantly for another 5 to 8 minutes until the onions are very aromatic.

- Add the mushrooms and cook, stirring frequently for another 5 minutes until the mushrooms brown slightly. Add the ground turkey and bison or beef and cook until meat is no longer pink but cooked through.

- Sprinkle the almond flour over the mixture, incorporating it evenly through the filling. Cook over low heat for another 5 minutes.

- Pour in the chicken stock and bring the mixture to a simmer for about 10 minutes or until the stock starts to thicken slightly. Spoon the filling into a three-quart, oven-safe casserole dish.

- To make the *Celery Root Mash*, add the garlic paste to the celery root. Mash together, adding coconut milk, ghee, or olive oil, ¼ teaspoon of garam masala, a pinch of cayenne, and sea salt and pepper to taste.

- When the mash is just the way you like it, spoon evenly on top of the filling and bake for 20 minutes. Serve immediately.

 CULINARY TERM: Garam Masala is a traditional aromatic spice blend that is widely used in Indian cooking. Garam masala means "warm or hot spices," and the concoction contains black peppercorns, cinnamon, cardamom, cloves, mace (or nutmeg) and cumin, as well as fennel and coriander. It adds potent flavor and zing to your dishes, and it also reportedly improves digestive fire, prevents cancer, wards off constipation, fights diabetes, and boosts overall health.

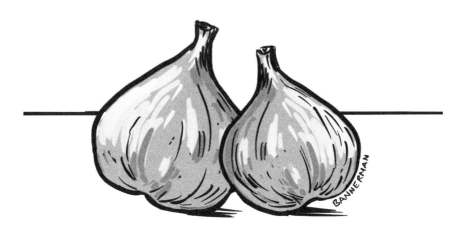

Pound-It-Out Chicken Cutlets
with Cilantro Pepita Verde Sauce
Serves 4

Ingredients

1 tablespoon oregano

1½ teaspoons chili powder

½ teaspoon ground cumin

¼ teaspoon ground cinnamon

½ teaspoon Himalayan sea salt

¼ teaspoon freshly cracked black pepper

½ cup almond flour

4 boneless, skinless chicken breasts

¼ cup avocado oil

Cilantro Pepita Verde Sauce
(see recipe on page 302)

3 tablespoons toasted pepita seeds for garnish

3 tablespoons chopped cilantro for garnish

Directions

Preheat the oven to 350°F.

- Cut parchment paper into 3 to 4 (12" × 12") sheets for pounding chicken.

- Line a rimmed baking sheet with parchment paper.

- Combine the oregano, chili powder, cumin, cinnamon, Himalayan sea salt, pepper, and almond flour in a Mason jar. Cap the jar securely and shake seasonings together. Set aside.

- Trim any fat from the chicken breasts and set aside on a large plate.

- Working with one piece at a time, lay a chicken breast on the cutting board. Place a sheet of parchment paper over the chicken, and with the smooth side of a meat pounder, mallet, or small frying pan, pound to flatten it. Have fun with this part!

- When the chicken breast is uniformly flattened to about ¼-inch thick, remove the parchment paper and place the breast on the prepared baking sheet. Repeat with the remaining chicken breasts, using a different piece of parchment paper each time. Discard the used parchment paper immediately and wash your hands thoroughly in hot soapy water.

- Pour the seasoned almond flour into a rectangular baking dish or pie pan. Coat each chicken breast thoroughly with the seasoned flour.

- Gently shake off any excess flour and place chicken back on the prepared baking sheet.

- Heat a ceramic-lined nonstick, or well-seasoned cast iron pan, over medium high heat. Add the avocado oil and swirl the pan around to coat the bottom of the pan evenly.

- When the pan is hot but not smoking, add the chicken breasts and cook undisturbed for 5 minutes. The chicken will easily come up from pan if allowed to brown. If it sticks slightly, give it a little nudge with tongs or a metal spatula and then flip over. If it doesn't lift away from the pan, it probably isn't browned enough.

Sometimes it sticks, so give the pan a shake but resist the urge to peel chicken from the pan.

- Once the chicken is lightly browned on both sides, return it to the baking sheet, making sure each chicken breast is evenly spaced apart. When all chicken breasts are browned and on the baking sheet, bake for 10 to 15 minutes or until a meat thermometer inserted in thickest part of chicken reads 165°F.

- While the chicken is baking, make the *Cilantro Pepita Verde Sauce*. To serve, spoon two tablespoons of sauce over chicken and top with the toasted pepitas and cilantro.

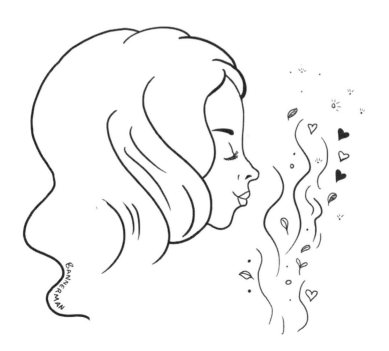

Cilantro Pepita Verde Sauce

Yield: ¾ cup

Ingredients

¼ cup pepita seeds

1 cup cilantro

3 tablespoons lime Juice

¼ teaspoon ground coriander

¼ cup extra-virgin olive oil

¼ teaspoon of, Himalayan sea salt

Freshly cracked black pepper, to taste

¼ cup water or enough to make sauce a pourable consistency

Directions

- Heat a dry skillet over low heat and add the pepitas. Shake the pan slightly to distribute seeds across pan. As they cook, the seeds will start to pop and turn lightly brown. They will smell very aromatic.

- Once the seeds are toasted, pour onto a cold plate to cool.

- Add the pepitas, cilantro, lime juice, ground coriander, olive oil, Himalayan sea salt, ground pepper, and water into a blender and purée until smooth.

 STORAGE POINTERS: *Store leftover Cilantro Pepita Verde Sauce in a Mason jar or airtight glass container and refrigerate for up to three days. Sauce can be used as a salad dressing or to flavor vegetables, fish, or meat.*

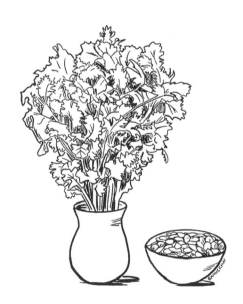

Savory-and-Sublime Spicy Miso Beef Stew

Serves 4

Ingredients

1 pound cubed beef stew meat

1 teaspoon Himalayan sea salt

3 tablespoons avocado oil or ghee, divided

1 small red onion, diced

2 carrots, medium, diced

1 celery stalk, small, diced

1½ cups shiitake mushrooms, sliced

¼ cup Bragg Liquid Aminos

2 tablespoons red or brown miso paste

1 teaspoon freshly cracked black pepper

2 teaspoon chili flakes, ground into a coarse powder, optional

2 tablespoons filtered water

2 cups shredded cabbage (green, purple, or Napa)

½ cup thinly sliced scallions (about 4)

3 cups *Bountiful Bone Broth* (see recipe on page 270) **or buy good quality, unsweetened, store-bought chicken stock or bone broth**

Himalayan sea salt, to taste

Directions

- Sprinkle each beef cube evenly with Himalayan sea salt. Follow instructions for pressure cooking in the Instant Pot® user's manual. Set Instant Pot to "Sauté High Heat" and add oil or ghee. If you don't have an Instant Pot, heat a heavy-bottomed pot over high heat and add the oil or ghee. Proceed with the recipe.

- Brown the beef on all sides in batches and transfer to a baking dish or pan. Set aside. Add remaining oil or ghee and cook onions, carrots, and celery while stirring frequently until the onions become translucent and softened.

- Add the shiitake mushrooms and continue to cook, stirring constantly until mushrooms are browned. Deglaze pan with Bragg Liquid Aminos. Scrape up the browned bits on the bottom of the pan with a wooden spoon and incorporate into cooked vegetables.

- In a small bowl, stir the miso, pepper, and chili flakes (if using) with water. Stir the mixture into vegetables, coating thoroughly. Add the cabbage, followed by beef, and top with half the scallions. Pour in the bone broth or chicken stock.

- Cover the Instant Pot and set to "Pressure Cook" for 25 minutes. If cooking on the stovetop, bring the stew to a boil, lower the heat to medium low, cover the pot, and simmer for 2½ hours or until beef comes apart easily when pierced with a fork.

- Use the "Natural Release" method once stew is finished. Season to taste with sea salt and pepper. Serve in bowls and garnish with remaining scallions.

Wild Roasted Salmon with Mustard Horseradish Butter
Serves 4

Ingredients

1 pound wild-caught salmon fillet, preferably king or coho salmon

1 heaping tablespoon ghee

2 teaspoons Dijon mustard

1 teaspoon prepared horseradish paste

Pinch of Himalayan sea salt

Pinch of freshly cracked pepper

Directions

Preheat the oven to 350°F.

- Remove any pin bones from the salmon fillet using tweezers and cut into 4 equal pieces. Place salmon pieces in a heat-proof glass baking pan. Melt the ghee and stir in the mustard and horseradish until sauce is emulsified (looks smooth and glossy). Season with a pinch each of Himalayan sea salt and freshly cracked pepper.

- Using a brush or back of a spoon, spread the mixture evenly onto each salmon piece.

- Roast for 15 to 20 minutes or until the salmon flakes easily with a fork.

 COOKING TIP: *You can roast the salmon with other dressings and sauces such as the Almond Ginger Turmeric Dressing or the Cilantro Pepita Verde Sauce. Brush the salmon generously with sauce or dressing of your choice and roast as directed in the Wild Roasted Salmon recipe.*

Keeping your body healthy is an expression of gratitude to the whole cosmos—the trees, the clouds, everything.[14]

—Thich Nhất Hanh (1926–2022), Vietnamese Buddhist monk, peace activist, and author

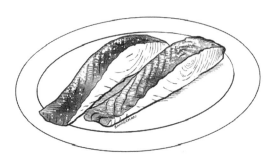

DESSERTS

We're delighted to present one recipe each week of the Bounce Back Diet for a healthy, delectable, KetoMod dessert.

 COACH CONNIE RECOMMENDS

These nutrient-packed, keto-friendly treats are especially yummy. Since your goal is to continue to shed weight and improve your health, enjoy just one serving. Get leftovers out of your home as soon as possible. Give the rest to your family, friends, neighbors, or coworkers.

The reason you want to have only one serving is because storing desserts in the fridge or freezer may be too tempting for some of you.

Years ago, after I triumphed over my own food issues and began to coach many carb and sugar addicts, I discovered the fastest and easiest way to keep eating healthy.

It's incredibly simple: *never ever* keep any tempting dishes—no matter how healthy they are—under your roof. That's why you'll get all these tasty leftover desserts out of sight, and hence, out of mind. A healthy nudge such as this will keep you on track.

Chocolate Spice Coconut Crunch Truffles

Yield: Approximately 6 round truffles
Serving size: 2 truffles

Ingredients

½ **cup unsweetened cacao powder**

¼ **teaspoon ground cinnamon**

¼ **teaspoon ginger**

⅛ **teaspoon cardamom**

⅛ **teaspoon Himalayan sea salt**

2 **tablespoons coconut oil, melted**

2 **tablespoons coconut butter, melted**

¼ **cup coconut cream* (the thick cream from a can of full-fat, unsweetened coconut milk)**

¼ **teaspoon vanilla powder or extract**

2 **tablespoons unsweetened shredded coconut**

Other topping options:

Cocoa nibs

Orange zest

Crushed toasted almonds

Crushed freeze-dried raspberries

Directions

- In the bowl of a food processor or blender, pulse the cacao powder with the cinnamon, ginger, cardamom, and Himalayan sea salt. Add the melted coconut oil, coconut butter, coconut cream, and vanilla. Process until the mixture is smooth.

- Transfer the mixture to a bowl and place in the freezer for 15 minutes or until it's firm enough to roll into truffles.

- While the truffle mixture is chilling, toast coconut in a dry skillet. Put toasted coconut onto a plate and set aside.

- Take the truffle mixture out of the freezer and roll into balls about ½ to 1 inch in diameter. Roll each truffle into toasted coconut or other optional toppings.

- Store the truffles in an airtight container in the refrigerator. Before serving, allow the truffles to come to room temperature for the best flavor and texture.

 COOKING TIP: *To thicken the consistency of the cream in a can of full-fat, unsweetened coconut milk, refrigerate it overnight.*

Lemon Coconut Cream Bon-Bons

Yield: Approximately 6 bon-bons
Serving size: 2 bon-bons

Ingredients

⅓ cup coconut butter

¼ cup coconut oil

¼ cup full-fat, unsweetened coconut milk

1 teaspoon lemon juice

1 tablespoon fresh lemon zest

1 teaspoon vanilla powder or vanilla bean seeds

Pinch of Himalayan sea salt

Directions

▪ Add the coconut butter, coconut oil, and coconut milk to a small saucepan. Melt together over low heat.

▪ When the mixture is melted, add the lemon juice, zest, vanilla, and sea salt. Taste and adjust flavors by adding more lemon juice, zest, vanilla, or sea salt.

▪ Pour the mixture into ice cube trays and freeze for an hour or until set. Remove bon-bons from the tray and place into a glass storage container with a lid and keep in refrigerator.

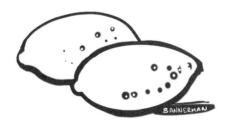

Coconut Vanilla Panna Cotta with Toasted Coconut

Yield: 1½ cups

Serving size: 3 (½ cup) portions

Ingredients

2 tablespoons filtered water

2 teaspoons powdered gelatin

1½ cups full-fat, unsweetened coconut milk

1 vanilla bean, seeds scraped, bean pod reserved or teaspoon of vanilla extract.

1 teaspoon lemon juice

¼ teaspoon Himalayan sea salt

2 tablespoons unsweetened coconut flakes, toasted

2 teaspoons pomegranate arils (seeds) or 3 raspberries per serving, for garnish

Directions

- Pour the water into a bowl; sprinkle the gelatin over the top and stir in gently until smooth. Set aside.

- Combine the coconut milk, vanilla bean seeds and the bean pod (or vanilla extract) into a small heavy saucepan. Stir over low heat until the coconut milk begins to simmer.

- Remove the saucepan from the heat and add the gelatin, stirring until it dissolves. Add the lemon juice and sea salt and allow the mixture to cool for 15 minutes.

- Divide the mixture among four small custard cups or jelly jars and cover with cheesecloth or beeswax wrap. Allow to set in the refrigerator for up to 6 hours or overnight. To serve, top each panna cotta with toasted coconut flakes and pomegranate arils or 3 raspberries.

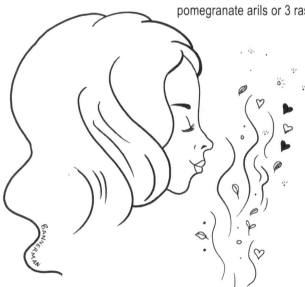

Conclusion

As fleeting commitments, diets often fail.
Thinking of dietary choices as part of who you are . . .
can give them real staying power.[1]

—**Nir Eyal**, bestselling author of *Indistractable*

FUEL YOUR ADVENTURE WITH FUN, FEASTS, AND FULFILLMENT

The most effective way to change your habits is to focus not on what you want to achieve, but on who you wish to become.[2]

—**James Clear**, author of the *New York Times* bestselling book
*Atomic Habits: An Easy & Proven Way
to Build Good Habits & Break Bad Ones*

Hurrah! You did it! You've kickstarted your adventure to prioritize your health, drop excess pounds while you heal your heart, and Bounce Back Boldly. You've set in motion a powerful process of transformation.

Think Positive and Ignore Pessimistic "Diets Don't Work" Predictions

At this point, let me prepare you. Cynics may cross your path. They may predict that you'll gain back all the weight you shed. Hold on! Please disregard those dismal predictions.

Yes, let's dispense with disheartening research, which suggests that 75 percent to 80 percent of people who initially peeled off a substantial amount of body fat may regain some or all of it within four to five years.[3]

Those fatalistic forecasts don't give you nearly enough credit. For starters, they don't look at the full picture. They don't take into account that you now understand why you ate badly and this knowledge is leading you to healthier behavior. They don't consider that you're choosing higher-quality, real foods instead of obsessively counting calories or carbs.

Finally, these negative people are clueless about the fact that you have an arsenal of powerful FEASTS (Fast, Easy, Awesome, Simple, Tested Strategies) and mindset-lifting DDEVA tactics (where you Desire, Decide, Expect, Visualize, and Affirm).

At this point, I urge you to instead consider hard-nosed research from scientists who discovered that ongoing weight loss and healthy maintenance is downright doable.

Yes, you can choose to discard unwanted excess weight and keep it off over the long term.

> *If you believe you can change—if you make it a habit—the change becomes real. This is the real power of habit: the insight that your habits are what you choose them to be. Once that choice occurs—and becomes automatic—it's not only real, it starts to seem inevitable.*[4]

—Charles Duhigg, Pulitzer Prize-winning journalist and author of the *New York Times* bestsellers, *The Power of Habit* and *Supercommunicators*

Studies Show You Can Keep Off the Pounds

It's now my pleasure to tell you about people who've successfully maintained their weight loss. We'll call them Successful Losers.

Perhaps the most promising results come from the National Weight Control Registry (NWCR), which has tracked more than 10,000 people—80 percent women and 20 percent men—who shed thirty pounds or more and kept them off one year or longer.[5] The average person melted away sixty-six pounds and stayed at the lower weight for 5.5 years.

The NWCR was founded in 1994 by obesity experts Rena Wing, PhD, professor of psychiatry and human behavior at Brown Medical School, and James O. Hill, PhD, professor of pediatrics and medicine at the University of Colorado Health Sciences Center.[6]

Their mission? To identify common characteristics and habits of "successful weight loss maintainers."

Replies from registry members reveal that the secret to keeping off the weight is to consistently practice several healthy behaviors:[7]

- 98 percent of Successful Losers modified their food intake with a low-fat or low-carb diet. (You're already curtailing carbs.)
- 90 percent exercise an hour a day on average—mostly walking. (Like them, you're moving every day.)
- 78 percent of NWCR members eat breakfast every morning. (Of course, you're doing that, too.)

- 75 percent weigh themselves at least once a week. (This is a good practice to keep.)
- 62 percent watch TV less than ten hours a week. (This is another smart habit that helps you sit less and move more.)

Now for more encouraging findings. Research shows that long-term weight maintenance gets easier over time. You read that right. *Easier.*

After tracking nearly 3,300 registry participants for ten years, researchers discovered that most Successful Losers remained at the lower weight for more than a decade, according to a study published in the *American Journal of Preventive Medicine.*[8]

In addition, Successful Losers in the registry maintained an average of 77 percent of their initial weight loss when followed up five years later. Ten years after coming on board, they had kept off 74 percent of their weight.

In the final analysis, participants in the National Weight Control Registry show that "people can successfully maintain substantial weight losses over a long-term follow-up, despite environmental and physiological challenges they may face," Dr. Wing explained to me.[9]

Bounce Back Boldly Weight Success Story

I lost fifty-two pounds in fifty-two weeks when I was fifty-two, and I've kept off every pound for 17 years. After a lifetime of struggling with sugar addiction, I was able to put in place the steps necessary to permanently remove the cravings from my life. I no longer eat any sweet food that contains sugar except for fresh fruit. That means no sugar, honey, maple syrup, agave nectar, or high fructose corn syrup. I also walk an hour a day, listening to music or audiobooks to keep myself motivated.[10]

—**Sue Brown,** National Weight Control Registry member, former sugar addict turned health coach, who now nurtures herself with yoga, gratitude, journaling, home cooking, Zumba, raw cacao nibs, and more

Successful Losers Found Their *Big Why*

We can learn more about what motivates people to remain at a healthier weight from a study in *Obesity* of more than 6,000 people, who shed more than fifty pounds on average and kept them off for more than five years while members of WW (formerly Weight Watchers).[11]

Those Successful Losers revealed the tremendous power of having a deep desire to succeed, or what we'll call a *Big Why*. For instance, participants were driven to success by health issues such as diabetes and heart conditions, pain, concerns about mobility, appearance, and suggestions from family or friends.

One weight maintainer, for instance, longed "to feel better" about herself. "I wasn't happy with how I looked or felt," she admitted.

Her Big Why? "I wanted to be happy, look good, and not be or feel limited in what I wore or what I did."

Those weight maintainers showed "perseverance in the face of setbacks," concluded Suzanne Phelan, PhD, who led the study. They regarded "setbacks as part of their successful journey. They were seen as a temporary interruption in their path."[12]

"Many weight-loss maintainers described getting back on track at the next meal or the next day and measuring overall success based on long-term goals," amplified Dr. Phelan, a professor in California Polytechnic State University's Department of Kinesiology and Public Health and director of the university's Center for Health Research.[13]

Thousands of successful role models have paved the way for you. They proved that you, too, can succeed when you're driven by your Big Whys.

Being fit and healthy is not about achieving the perfect body,
but about feeling strong, confident, and capable.[14]

—**AJ Jacobs**, author of the humorous, self-deprecating
New York Times bestseller *Drop Dead Healthy:*
One Man's Humble Quest for Bodily Perfection

Bounce Back Boldly Weight Success Story

Ultimately it came down to . . . deciding whether I wanted to advance toward the grave in a state of decrepit stupor, or rise and advance in life as a fresh, vital being, full of youthful energy and joy. . . . Losing weight and being healthy can be so simple and easy. Your goal should never be weight loss but rather to have true health and respect for the gift of life.[15]

—**Bryant McGill**, bestselling author of *Simple Reminders: Inspiration for Living Your Best Life* and thought leader, who shed more than 100 pounds and healed from seventeen health challenges, including heart disease, high blood pressure, and borderline diabetes

Remember to Let GoalPowerPlus Drive You to Feel Better

As you gear up to succeed, bear in mind that you don't need to rely on willpower (the ability to exert self-control) to resist short-term temptations (cookies, fast foods, or carbage). Instead, you're now unleashing GoalPowerPlus, which makes it much easier to stay in control.

But be on the lookout for naysayers who may suggest that you'll run out of willpower. They may have bought into the widely shared *ego-depletion theory* from social psychologist Roy Baumeister, PhD, who suggested that willpower is a limited resource that can get fatigued like a muscle when you overuse it.[16]

You now know better. Let me close this discussion of willpower by sharing promising results from two studies:

- **Your willpower or your ability to exercise self-control is contingent on what you believe to be true.** So suggested a study in *Psychological Science*. Researchers from Stanford University proposed that if you think you have available willpower, you do. As a result, you're more likely to achieve your goals and change unwanted behaviors.[17]

- **You'll be more successful at shedding weight when you're motivated by personal reasons versus external ones.** In other words, you're not driven by "perceived pressure from others and feelings of guilt," observed researchers for a study in the *Journal of Nutrition Education and Behavior*.[18]

Whether you aim to lose 20 pounds or you want to launch your own business, mental strength is the key to long-term success. After all, you need fierce determination and tenacity to reach your greatest potential.[19]

—**Amy Morin**, psychotherapist, social worker,
Northeastern University instructor, and author of the
bestseller *13 Things Mentally Strong People Don't Do*

Fill Your Journey with Fun and Pleasure

Now I need to debunk another oft-cited concern of people who go on a plan to fit into smaller-size clothes. You've probably heard of (or maybe you've been one of) those folks who wail and worry that they'll feel deprived while watching what they eat. Hogwash!

Doubtful dieters tend to focus on what foods are *off limits* rather than on what delicious foods are *on the menu*. That approach sucks the joy out of eating. Indeed, you get into trouble when you dwell on what foods *you can't have* rather than appreciating what *you can have*.

Soon, I predict, you'll continue to choose, consume, and enjoy quality foods and drinks *not* because of *how good you'll look*, but because of *how good you'll feel*. In fact, you'll find that eating better is downright transformational.

Healthy eating builds massive momentum. The more you pick nutritious foods, the more you'll want to continue to do so. All those top-quality bites contribute to bringing more joy, good health, and peace of mind into your life.

*Start valuing the health benefits and energy consequences of
the foods [you] eat as much or more than the taste.*[20]

—**Hal Elrod,** international keynote speaker and bestselling
author of *The Miracle Morning* and *The Miracle Equation*

Clean Food Is the Superhighway to Your Superpower

By now, I hope you realize that eating quality foods and shedding pounds
(whatever amount your doctor suggests) is a powerful way to kickstart
your awesome life. By upgrading your diet, you're upgrading your life.

Putting food in its proper place is powerful. When you eat better, you
feel better. When you eat better, you *live* better. When you eat better, you
are better.

Don't be fooled by the simplicity of this concept. Just ask those of us
who happily eat healthy foods most (if not all) the time. We intentionally
choose high-quality foods not because we should, but because we feel
great when we make top-notch choices.

What it comes down to is this: when you select superior foods, you're
giving yourself and your body lots of love. Admittedly, this may sound
somewhat hokey, but it's true. When you eat well, you're treasuring your
vessel, your health, and your life.

In the final analysis, nourishing yourself with top-notch foods is a fast
and sure-fire path to power, joy, and self-love.

Be Optimistic about Your Success

Now let's turn our attention to your attitude. Do you look at the glass
as half-empty or half-full? We'll now focus on fascinating research that
explores the benefits of optimism:

- **Taking an optimistic approach to weight loss yields better
  results.** Patients were more likely to participate in a recommended
  weight loss program and they shed more pounds if obesity was presented as an "opportunity." For the study in the *Annals of Internal
  Medicine*, researchers analyzed recordings from doctor-patient conversations and found that patients were more successful when their

physicians took an upbeat, "good news" approach that communicated positivity, optimism, and excitement; made little mention of obesity, weight, or BMI as a problem; and focused on the benefits of weight loss.[21]

- **You may eat better if you're optimistic.** Research in *Nutrition Journal* found that those who are optimists eat more healthy foods and do less snacking.[22]
- **Optimistic folks are healthier.** A study of more than 70,000 women in the *American Journal of Epidemiology* found that optimists had a significantly lower risk of dying from such diseases as heart disease, stroke, and cancer, as well as a better quality of life, lower rates of depression, and higher energy levels.[23]

There's no higher value than aspiring to be better tomorrow than we are today.[24]

—**Adam Grant**, organizational psychologist and # 1 *New York Times* bestselling author of *Hidden Potential* and *Think Again*

Start to Explore Your *Whats*

Before we part company, I want to remind you: This isn't just a diet book; it's a transformational guide. It's time to start thinking big.

In Part II, I invited you to focus on your *Whys* so you could discover the specific factors that led you to eat badly and blow your diet.

In Part III, you shifted gears and began to discover the *Hows* or FEASTS (Fast, Easy, Awesome, Simple, Tested Strategies) that can help you quickly step into your power, claim calm, and enjoy a vibrant you.

Now that you're well-nourished and practicing healthy habits, you want to think about your *Whats*.

Ask yourself, "What would I love?" Think bigger, bolder, and braver. Dream of what you would absolutely love, not asking how but only what.[25]

—**Mary Morrissey**, renowned expert on Dream Building and author of *Brave Thinking*

Celebrate like a Bounce Back Boldly Champion

As we wrap up our time together, take pride in all you've accomplished to ensure your success.

Let me put on my fairy godmother hat again. I now dub you a *Bounce Back Boldly Champion*.

You deserve high praise. You faced your challenges head on. You delved deep to discover why you ate badly. You're now selecting nutrient-rich foods, uplifting activities, and smart habits, all of which lay the groundwork for you to become a better you.

> *I have learned that champions aren't just born; champions can be made when they embrace and commit to life-changing positive habits.*[26]

—Lewis Howes, former pro football player, podcast host, and author of the *New York Times* bestselling book *The Greatness Mindset*

It's time to celebrate. Go to a private place where you can let loose. Stand tall. Triumphantly throw your hands up in the air.

Proudly proclaim, "Yes! I'm on my way! I'm doing it! Happier, healthier, stronger body, here I come!"

Now take that festive spirit into our fun-filled Dance Party together.

Raise your arms. Lift your legs. Swivel your hips. Now gyrate to these feel-good victory songs:

- "Don't Stop Believin'" from Journey[27]
- "Just the Way You Are" by Bruno Mars[28]
- "The Champion" by Carrie Underwood[29]
- "Dancing Queen" by ABBA[30]
- "Unstoppable" by Sia[31]

It's been a pleasure and an honor to be your guide as you jump-start your journey to peel off pounds, take back your power, and become a better, happier, healthier version of yourself.

Woo Hoo! You're on your way to Bounce Back Boldly.[32]

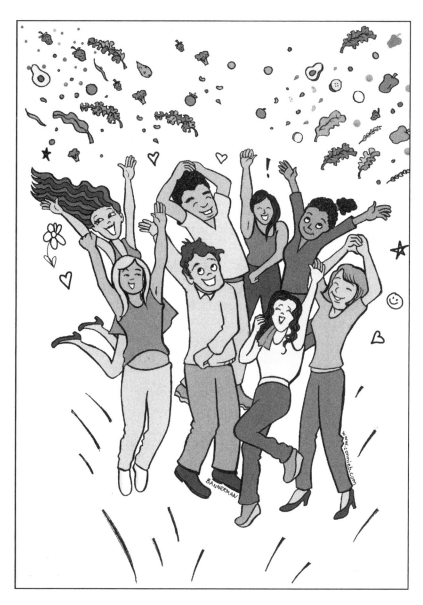

Sweet success is yours!

Recommended Resources

B elow you'll find a list of some of my favorite thought leaders, books, programs, and products, which can help you Bounce Back Boldly and lead a healthier, happier, more fulfilling life. To be fair, I've listed them alphabetically. Since I shared so many options, just choose those that feel like a good fit for you. You also can find this list online at www.connieb.com/Recommended-Resources.

Alpha-Stim: This painless, nondrug, FDA-cleared medical device is recommended by physicians, dentists, and other health care professionals to treat anxiety, insomnia, and depression, along with acute, chronic, or post-traumatic pain. Alpha-Stim is supported by more than 100 independent, controlled research studies and published reports. The first time I experienced the soothing effects of this portable device was at the dentist's office. When I felt so calm during dental surgery, I immediately bought my own gadget to use at home. www.alpha-stim.com

Bala Bangles: Now that you're exercising more, you can add resistance to your workouts using versatile, comfortable, weighted Bala Bangles and Bala Bars. www.shopbala.com/

BioMat: This cutting-edge wellness tool—which is used by thousands of medical doctors, physical therapists, acupuncturists, massage therapists, and other health and wellness professionals—features unique medical and therapeutic properties that are reportedly rooted in Nobel Prize-winning research and NASA's top-rated infrared technology. A BioMat harnesses the power of infrared, amethyst, and tourmaline crystals and negative ions. For my part, if I have back pain—even after doing Pilates, moving, or stretching—my BioMat always gives me relief within minutes. And great sleep, too. www.biomat.com

Brave Thinking Institute: This company—founded by motivational speaker, minister, personal development expert, and bestselling author Mary Morrissey—helps thousands of people worldwide see, feel, and achieve their dreams using a powerful manifestation process called Dream Building. www.bravethinkinginstitute.com

Brown, Brené, PhD: This research professor at the University of Houston Graduate College of Social Work and expert on shame, courage, vulnerability, and authenticity offers enlightening TED talks, *New York Times* bestselling books (*Rising Strong, Daring Greatly*, etc.), and the Netflix special *The Call to Courage*. www.brenebrown.com

Cain, Susan: If you're an introvert or close to someone who is, I urge you to read Cain's *New York Times* bestseller *Quiet: The Power of Introverts in a World That Can't Stop Talking*. As an introvert myself, this book was a game-changer for me. Her follow-up book, *Bittersweet: How Sorrow and Longing Make Us Whole*, is also transformative. www.susancain.net

Cameron, Julia: Even if you're not creative, Cameron can help awaken your imagination. Just follow guidelines she lays out in her bestselling book *The Artist's Way: A Spiritual Path to Higher Creativity*. www.juliacameronlive.com

Canfield, Jack: The coauthor of the mega-bestselling *Chicken Soup for the Soul* series shares valuable steps to help you accomplish your goals in his guide, *The Success Principles: How to Get from Where You Are to Where You Want to Be*. www.thesuccessprinciples.com

Clear, James: The author of the long-running #1 *New York Times* bestselling book *Atomic Habits: An Easy & Proven Way to Build Good Habits & Break Bad Ones*, shares practical information to help you create positive habits. www.JamesClear.com

Eco-Friendly Metal Food Containers: While you eat healthy foods, I urge you to do your part to protect our planet. Reduce waste into landfills by buying environmentally friendly, reusable metal food containers. Some vendors: www.ecolunchboxes.com, www.ecozoi.com, www.planetbox.com, and www.ukonserve.com.

Eco-Friendly Water Bottles: Save money and show love for Mother Earth by using reusable water bottles. A few sources: www.binkmade.com, www.ecovessel.com, www.hydroflask.com, www.kleankanteen.com, and www.puristcollective.com.

Emotional Freedom Technique (EFT) or Tapping: These are some resources to help you triumph over overeating, PTSD, grief, pain, anxiety, or other issues:

- **EFT Universe.** This community, spearheaded by Dr. Dawson Church, offers workshops, meditations, and a Be Trauma Free course. eftuniverse.com/

- **EFT Practitioners.** Find a trained practitioner by state, country, and specialty. www.eftuniverse.com/practitioners

- **Tapping Q&A.** Gene Monterastelli offers more than 500 free EFT resources, from the basics of how to tap to advanced tapping tools. www.tappingqanda.com

- **Tapping Solution, The.** Offers masterclasses, the annual Tapping World Summit, an app, and my favorite, the Tapping Insiders Club. www.thetappingsolution.com

- **Tap With Brad.** Brad Yates offers a new tapping video every week (more than 1,000 tap-along programs) on his YouTube.com channel. You may like his "I Need to Stuff My Face!" tapping sequence. www.tapwithbrad.com

- **Veterans Stress Solution (formerly Veterans Stress Project).** Free phone, online, or in-person EFT sessions are available to current military officers, veterans, and their family members to help those with PTSD get their lives back. www.stresssolution.org/provider-directory

EMF Blockers: To reduce harmful blue light, which can cause eye strain and disrupt your sleep, you can get eye-protecting blue-blockers from www.pixeleyewear.com, www.raoptics.com, www.swanwicksleep.com, and www.truedark.com.

EMF Protection: You may be able to protect yourself from harmful electromagnetic frequencies with products from www.airestech.com, www.defendershield.com, www.emfblues.com, www.emf-harmony.com, and www.HarmoniPendant.com.

Essential Oils: These are bottled plant extracts, which are made by steaming or pressing plants. The fragrant aromas may provide healing properties and help with stress, insomnia, or pain. Some sources: www.YoungLiving.com, www.Doterra.com, and www.planttherapy.com.

Exercise Classes Online: If you'd like to work out at home, here are some great options:

- Blogilates (www.blogilates.com)
- The Fitness Marshall (www.thefitnessmarshall.org)
- Flipping 50 (www.flippingfifty.com)
- Jenny McClendon (www.jennyfitstart.com)
- Lucy Wyndham-Read (www.lwrfitness.com)
- Pilatesology (www.pilatesology.com)
- Walk at Home (www.walkathome.com), and
- Yoga with Adriene (www.yogawithadriene.com).

For more details, see www.connieb.com/exercise-classes-online

Green Building Supply: If you own your home, you may wish to get nontoxic, sustainable, ecofriendly flooring products, paints, and other products. www.greenbuildingsupply.com

Hay House: The largest publisher of transformational programs and books, Hay House is home to such influencers as Gabrielle Bernstein, Dr. Joe Dispenza, and the pioneering Louise Hay, whose book *You Can Heal Your Life* sold more than fifty million copies. www.hayhouse.com

Healthy Food & Beverages:

- **Bone Broth Vendors.** For a list of companies that offer organic, gluten-free frozen or powdered bone broth, see my blog post at www.connieb.com/where-to-buy-quality-bone-broth.

- **Brands and Vendors We Like.** To find companies that offer sugar-free, gluten-free, dairy-free, organic products, turn to page 231 or visit www.connieb.com/healthy-food-resources.

- **Farmers' Markets.** To find a farmers' market near you, enter your zip code into the USDA's directory at https://www.ams.usda.gov/local-food-directories/farmersmarkets.

- **Healthy but "Ugly" Real Foods.** Save money when you buy excess, unusual-shaped healthy foods that would otherwise be thrown into landfills just because they're "ugly." All foods will be shipped directly to you. Check out www.imperfectfoods.com or www.misfitsmarket.com.

- **Herbal Teas.** You can get fruity, savory, floral, earthy, sweet, sugar-free herbal teas from www.adagio.com, www.artoftea.com, www.goodearth.com, www.organicindia.com, www.tazo.com, www.traditionalmedicinals.com, and www.yogitea.com.

- **CSAs:** Find a nearby Community-Supported Agriculture, or CSA, whose members weekly get reasonably priced, full or half-shares of seasonal, locally sourced veggies, eggs, meats, poultry, fruit, flowers, and herbs from a specific farm or group of farms in their region. www.localharvest.org/csa

- **Thrive Market.** This e-commerce, membership-based retailer offers high-quality natural, organic food products at reduced prices. If you like, while checking out, you can donate your savings to charity. www.thrivemarket.com

Hyman, Mark, MD: The renowned integrative physician, *New York Times* bestselling author (of *Eat Fat, Get Thin*, etc.), and podcast host (*The Dr. Hyman Show*) shares a wealth of valuable information. www.drhyman.com

Insight Timer: You can access more than 150,000 meditations from psychologists, spiritual leaders, and mindfulness teachers on this app for sleep, anxiety, and stress. www.insighttimer.com

Lamott, Anne: The compassionate, self-deprecating, humorous writer will entertain you with such bestsellers as *Somehow*; *Almost Everything*; *Hallelujah Anyway*; *Small Victories*; and *Help, Thanks, Wow*. It's fun listening to Anne read her books. www.facebook.com/AnneLamott

McColl, Peggy: This manifestation expert, "Prosperity Mentor," and author of the *Savvy Wisdom* trilogy, offers various programs to authors, experts, and entrepreneurs. I especially like Peggy's innovative Club Achieve program, where we study transformational books every weekday morning for up to half an hour. www.peggymccoll.com

Milkman, Katy, PhD: Behavioral scientist, economist, author of *How to Change*, and cofounder/codirector of the Behavior Change for Good Initiative shares great info about "fresh starts," "temptation bundling," and other smart practices to beat procrastination, exercise more, etc. www.katymilkman.com

Mindvalley: This innovative personal transformation learning platform offers many cutting-edge courses (called Quests) on such topics as meditation, abundance, entrepreneurship, performance, fitness, health, and relationships. You may want to begin with the Silva Ultramind System and the Be Extraordinary Quests programs taught by Mindvalley founder/entrepreneur Vishen Lakhiani. www.mindvalley.com

Mindfulness Meditation: To get guided meditation programs, see a list of resources at my blog at www.connieb.com/Mindfulness-Meditation-Resources.

Mind Movies: This is a great tool to help you easily visualize the great health, body, and life you'd love. With Mind Movies, you create and watch three-to-five-minute videos, complete with positive affirmations, invigorating music, and powerful images, which show you having already achieved your goals. Meanwhile, Mind Movies Matrix adds brain-wave entrainment and subliminal messages to Mind Movies to retrain your brain for success. Both programs come from entrepreneurs Natalie Ledwell and Glen Ledwell. www.mindmovies.com

Moss, Michael: To get more insights about how the food industry may have caused you to become addicted to sugary, fatty, salty junk foods, read *Salt Sugar Fat* and/or *Hooked* from investigative journalist Michael Moss. www.mossbooks.us/

MyNeuroGym: Provides Winning the Game of (Weight Loss, Business, Procrastination, etc.) trainings that use science-based methods to help you recognize and release mental or emotional obstacles that retrain your brain for success. Founded by entrepreneur and mindset teacher John Assaraf. My Accountability Buddy Emily Johnson and I are still going strong after 900 days and counting. www.myneurogym.com.

Olympic State of Mind: Watch videos of Olympians performing dazzling athletic feats and learn how sports psychology techniques of Olympic winners can help you have an "Olympic State of Mind." www.olympics.com/en/original-series/olympic-state-of-mind/

Pilates Machine: The Wunda Chair is my favorite piece of home workout equipment. In addition to working out on it twice a week with my trainer, I take quick breaks on it to stretch my back, strengthen my core, and build my muscles. https://www.gratzpilates.com/products/wunda-chair/

Primal Life Organics: Health expert Trina Felber, RN, created nontoxic, chemical-free, sustainable products such as organic toothpowder, a natural teeth-whitening system, and healthy deodorant. www.primallifeorganics.com

Robbins, Mel: The #1 ranking and Webby award-winning podcaster (*The Mel Robbins Podcast*) and bestselling author (*The Let Them Theory, The High 5 Habit*, and *The 5 Second Rule*) offers many powerful, proven, science-backed tools to help you become confident, effective, and fulfilled. If you'd like to be motivated, Mel can do it magnificently. While I was wrapping up this book, I took Mel's life-changing, empowering, innovative, six-month LAUNCH course. www.MelRobbins.com

Social Dilemma, The: This eye-opening Netflix documentary features top experts sounding the alarm on the dangerous potential of overdoing social networking. www.thesocialdilemma.com

Standing Desk: To move more and sit less, I recommend getting a height-adjustable desk if you can. The one I use and love is a Jarvis bamboo desk. www.fully.com

Stickk: This innovative program uses lessons from behavioral economics to help people achieve personal goals through commitment contracts. It was founded by academics who've extensively studied commitment contracts. www.stickk.com

The Oprah Podcast: The renowned host Oprah Winfrey talks with today's foremost thought leaders, global newsmakers, bestselling authors, and visionaries. The show explores themes such as happiness, resilience, consciousness, and connection. Every month, she interviews authors for "Oprah's Book Club Presented by Starbucks" in front of live audiences at Starbucks across the country. *The Oprah Podcast* is available on Apple, Spotify or wherever you listen to podcasts.

The Universe Talks (TUT): Mike Dooley, a motivating metaphysical teacher, entrepreneur, and *New York Times* bestselling author, offers a variety of reasonably priced courses that help you achieve your goals, including the 7-Day Creative Visualization Adventure. www.tut.com

Virgin, JJ: The celebrity nutrition expert, Fitness Hall of Famer, and *New York Times* bestselling author hosts the *Well Beyond 40 with JJ Virgin* podcast, which helps women over forty lose fat, drop inflammation, age powerfully by healing their metabolism, and prevent weight regain. www.jjvirgin.com

Vision Boards: Here are some resources to help you create your own vision board: www.canva.com/create/vision-boards/, www.dreambigcollection.com, and www.picmonkey.com/design/vision-board-maker.

Water Filters: Now that you're drinking ample water, consider getting a countertop water filter to remove impurities. Some ideas: www.aquatruwater.com, www.berkeyfilters.com (travel size available), www.bluevua.com, www.brita.com, and www.rkin.com.

Yoloha Yoga: When I searched for a healthy yoga mat that wasn't made of smelly polyvinyl chloride (PVC), I was excited to find this healthy alternative. Yoloha's yoga mats, blocks, cushions, and wheels are all made of sustainable, natural materials and organic cork. www.yolohayoga.com

You Are a Badass **(Books):** Self-described "motivational cattle prod" Jen Sincero is author of the fun, inspiring *Badass* books, including the #1 *New York Times* bestseller, *You Are a Badass: How to Stop Doubting Your Greatness and Start Living an Awesome Life.* I love listening to Sincero read her cleverly written books to help you fire up your badassery. www.jensincero.com

Endnotes
(Where You'll Find Them)

Initially, this section was supposed to run at the back of the physical book. But when the detailed list of notes, references, and peer-reviewed scientific papers filled 98 pages (using tiny print), it made sense to move the endnotes to my website to save paper, shorten the book to a manageable size, and lower your cost to purchase this book.

To complete this labor-intensive endnotes project, I received invaluable assistance from the dedicated Mckenzie Maira and Melissa Boles, who carefully verified facts, double-checked URLs, and organized hundreds of citations according to our modified *Chicago Manual of Style* format. Special thanks also go to Kaitlyn Arford and Lillian Kennedy.

Although we fastidiously checked all references, URLs for scientific studies and blog posts may change over time. Therefore, you may find an expired link. That's where you come in. If you find a citation that needs to be updated or corrected, please let me know so I can fix it on my website. To reach me, just hit the contact link on my website, www.connieb.com. Make sure to specify "Endnotes correction" in the subject line.

Now, to see the thousands of sources for this book, visit www.connieb.com/i-blew-my-diet-now-what/endnotes. I will continue to update the Endnotes as new information becomes available.

Beyond-the-Book Support

Access all gifts to enhance your reading experience
at www.BounceBackDiet.com/Book-Bonuses.

Blog Posts

1. Where to Find a Nutrition-Savvy Doctor
   www.connieb.com/Where-to-Find-a-Nutrition-Savvy-Doctor

2. Where to Get Grief Support
   www.connieb.com/Where-to-Get-Grief-support

3. Mindfulness Meditation Resources
   www.connieb.com/Mindfulness-Meditation-Resources

4. Where to Buy Quality Bone Broth
   www.connieb.com/Where-to-Buy-Quality-Bone-Broth

5. Popular Online Workouts
   www.connieb.com/Popular-Online-Workouts

6. Healthy Snacks to Pack
   www.connieb.com/Healthy-Snacks-to-Pack

7. Recommended Resources
   www.connieb.com/Recommended-Resources

Index

Recipe Index

Entries for recipes are shown as **bold** page numbers.

Join Me: Donate to the Hypoglycemia Support Foundation

The Hypoglycemia Support Foundation (HSF) educates people about the causes, prevention, and management of the often-misunderstood condition of low blood sugar, which affects millions of people worldwide.

The HSF was founded in 1980 by the visionary patient advocate Roberta Ruggiero, who has helped thousands of desperate people who seek to feel better when they finally discover or suspect that they have reactive hypoglycemia.

The Hypoglycemia Support Foundation—led by the insightful CEO Wolfram Alderson—has spearheaded numerous worthwhile projects, including the infographic, "Are You on the Blood Sugar Rollercoaster?," which helps patients in their time of need.

The HSF also has partnered with cutting-edge organizations and world-renowned physicians, including the acclaimed neuroendocrinologist Dr. Robert Lustig (bestselling author of *Fat Chance* and *Metabolical*) to help people—not just with hypoglycemia but with prediabetes and type 2 diabetes—navigate a food supply that is flooded with added sugars.

The HSF also has many other exciting programs in the works to help both physicians and their patients.

Wondering why I picked this charity to invite you to support? Because I'm one of those very grateful folks who've benefited greatly from the HSF's invaluable support. Thanks to this organization's vital guidance, I now thrive and easily manage this condition.

It's now time for me to give back, which is why I'm gratefully donating a percentage of book sales to this remarkable charity. If you can, please join me.

To support the Hypoglycemia Support Foundation's valuable work, go here: www.hypoglycemia.org/donate.

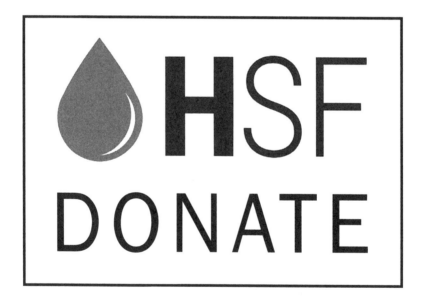

Acknowledgments

This book is finally seeing the light of day after more than seven years of research, rumination, and literary gestation. While taking this idea-to-book journey, I've been honored to have dozens of astute, creative, accomplished people in my corner.

First, my unwavering appreciation goes to the amazing authors' guru Steve Harrison for this book's clever title, *I Blew My Diet! Now What?*

To help me get this book into publishable shape, I'm greatly indebted to the amiable, fast-working, big-picture editor Sydny Miner, who expeditiously swept in to provide many recommendations to make this book flow, read, and serve you better.

Meanwhile, during this book's lengthy development phase, I was thankful to be guided by experienced book editor Nancy Hancock. Among other things, Nancy helped me identify which angles to pursue so readers get the help they need.

As for talented recipe formulators Lizette and Geoff Marx, they deserve a gleeful "Wow!" for diligently creating, testing, and rechecking their original KetoMod recipes.

Next, I owe enormous gratitude to the talented Pete Garceau for the stunning cover design, Isabella Bannerman for the entertaining cartoons, and Adept Content Solutions for the dazzling interior.

Now we come to my most remarkable mentors. Thank you a million, Mary Morrissey, John Assaraf, Mel Robbins, Mike Dooley, Natalie Ledwell, Jack Canfield, Gabrielle Bernstein, Peggy McColl, Tony Robbins, Jen Sincero, and Marci Shimoff for helping me boost my mindset, tune into infinite wisdom, adopt empowering practices, and dream big.

Since this book required massive amounts of research, I'm beholden to the accomplished journalists Jill Waldbieser, Angela Dowden, Lisa Milbrand, Alexandra Frost, Amanda Loudin, Gary Krebs, Ron Motta, Jill Neimark, Randy Fitzgerald, Cindy Pearlman, Michelle G. Sullivan, Malcolm Nicholl, and Susan Karlin. They all helped me find and make sense of hundreds of relevant, cutting-edge, evidence-based studies, which shed light on this book's many subjects. Likewise, I'm grateful to Susan Shapiro, Sam Horn, Gerry Jonas, Julia Pastore, Stephanie Abarbanel, "Book Mama" Linda Sivertsen, Roger Love, Daren LaCroix, Chris McGuire, and TEDxSanDiego.

Moreover, I especially appreciate the scientific researchers and experts who took time to answer my many questions. Special thanks, in particular, go to Dr. Peta Stapleton, Dr. Srini Pillay, Dr. Rena Wing, Professor Jackie Andrade, Mark Robert Waldman, Dr. Matthew Lieberman, Dr. Suzanne Phelan, Dr. Serge Ahmed, Dr. Jason Fanning, Professor Bärbel A. Knäuper, Dr. Christopher Cascio, Dr. Janet Polivy, Dr. David Ludwig, Dr. Dawson Church, and Dr. David Feinstein.

For this, my third book, I had the exciting and empowering experience of working with a hybrid publisher instead of a traditional publisher as I did for my first two books. It's been a joy to work with Adrianna Hernandez, Dee Kerr, Tanya Hall, Madison Johnson, and other awesome people at the Greenleaf Book Group while I exercised more creative control to make this the best book possible.

Meanwhile, I'm grateful to savvy publishing gurus Reid Tracy and Kelly Notaras for the Hay House Authorpreneur program. Many thanks also go to my literary agent Bill Gladstone of Waterside Productions for his continued support. (May you RIP.) I'm also grateful to Ken Browning, the Independent Book Publishers Association, the Nonfiction Authors Association, and the Authors Guild for their invaluable services. Thankful nods also go to Cindy Watson, Kathi Dunn, Scott Halford, Brooke Warner, Wendy Wong, Nicole Vazquez, and Rhoni Blankenhorn.

As for book marketing, publicity, and launching, I was happy to learn from and lean on the talented, knowledgeable Ashley Sandberg and the incredible team at Triple 7 Public Relations, as well as Shannon McCaffery, John Kremer, Jane Friedman, Danette Kubanda, Nick Suma, Bill Harrison,

Gina Callaway, and Olga Nieuwenhuizen. I also received instrumental guidance from Ray Edwards, Chris Winfield, Jen Gottlieb, Paula Rizzo, Joel Roberts, Jeff Walker, Ryan Levesque, John Lee Dumas, Tim Grahl, Jordan McAuley, Pat Flynn, John Boggs, and David Friedman.

My heartfelt appreciation also goes to the motivating thought leaders and authors Susan Cain, Dr. Katy Milkman, Dr. Angela Duckworth, Dr. Brené Brown, Dr. Amy Cuddy, Anne Lamott, Hal Elrod, Elizabeth Gilbert, and Cheryl Strayed.

Likewise, I'm indebted to Kris Carr, Pam Grout, Katherine Schwarzenegger, Cheryl Richardson, Dr. Mark Hyman, Dr. Daniel Amen, Dr. David Perlmutter, Dr. Jon Kabat-Zinn, Michael Moss, Gary Taubes, Dr. Sanjay Gupta, Michael Pollan, Dr. Christiane Northrup, Ocean Robbins, and Tim Ferriss. Grateful nods also go to the late legends Bob Proctor, Louise Hay, and Dr. Wayne Dyer.

More kudos are due to gifted speaking trainers Lisa Nichols, Bo Eason, Lisa Sasevich, Lynn Rose, Sean Smith, Pete Vargas III, Pat Quinn, Geoffrey Berwind, Chris Smith, Kymberlee Weil, Dr. Mark Tager, Robert John Hughes, Victoria Labalme, as well as Michael and Amy Port.

Furthermore, I appreciate JJ Virgin for creating the Mindshare Collaborative for us health and wellness professionals. I'm particularly grateful to Mary Agnes Antonopoulos, Michael and Izabella Wentz, Magdalena Wszelaki, Michele Drielick, and Karl Krummenacher for their pivotal tips or referrals.

More thanks go to Arielle Ford, Marie Forleo, Amy Porterfield, Brendon Burchard, Michael Hyatt, Chalene Johnson, Mari Smith, Tana Amen, David Wolfe, Sean Croxton, Bill Barren, Mastin Kipp, Mark Sisson, Sage Lavine, Allison Melody, Christian Mickelsen, Marla Cilley, Mandy Morris, Oliver Nino, Jim Padilla, Kim Nishida, Christie Turley, Michelle Pariza Wacek, Greg Jacobson, Muni Syed, Mike Koenigs, Doug Reynolds, Greg Reid, and Dave Jackson.

As for my own Bounce Back Boldly journey, I'm deeply grateful to Dr. Kistin Neff, Dr. Chris Germer, Dr. Ken Druck, David Asprey and 40 Years of Zen, Dr. Diana Pickett, David Kessler, Becki Hawkins, Deepak Chopra, Dr. Mary Ayers, Debora Wayne, Dr. Bernie Siegel, Dr. Jacob Teitelbaum, Kirsten Welles, Deborah Brenner-Liss, Dr. Joan Rosenberg, Carol Look, Dr. George Pratt, Amorah Kelly, David Rourke, Michael Nitti, David Hipshman, Zack Pelzel, Michelle Vandepass, Debra Artura, and Beata Booth.

On a lighter note, I'm laugh-out-loud grateful to *The Late Show with Stephen Colbert* for cracking me up often while I was completing this book during our world's challenging times.

I've also appreciated being entertained and educated weekdays by *The View* co-hosts Whoopi Goldberg, Sonny Hostin, Joy Behar, Sara Haines, Ana Navarro, and Alyssa Farah Griffin.

Now I need to share "You're awesome!" raves to my stalwart supporters Cassy Da Silva, Dr. Jill Baron, Dr. Keith Berkowitz, Roberta Ruggiero, and Betsy Rosenberg. Many, many, many thanks also go to my dedicated, always-supportive, motivational Accountability Buddies Emily Johnson and Jelayne Miles.

If I've inadvertently left out anyone who inspired me or gave me important information over the years, I apologize. Please know that I greatly appreciate you.

Finally, to you, dear reader, thank you for spending your precious time with me. I hope that this book gives you the information, insights, and guidance you need to take back your power, shed excess weight while eating quality foods, and step into your best life.

Connie Bennett

Connie Bennett
October 16, 2024

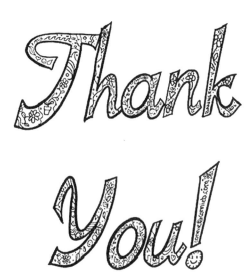

About The Author
CONNIE BENNETT

C onnie Bennett is an empowering, enthusiastic, experienced journalist and author of the bestselling books *Sugar Shock!* and *Beyond Sugar Shock.* A former carb and sugar addict, Connie is now a passionate clean-foods advocate, healthy-living aficionado, thought leader, DreamBuilder® Coach, certified health coach, life coach, EFT practitioner, motivational speaker, and champion of proven, powerful science-based tools to transform setbacks into breakthroughs.

Connie has been featured by hundreds of media outlets, including *CBS News Sunday Morning, Oprah & Friends Radio, The Howard Stern Show, TIME, Woman's World, Women's Weekly, The Library Journal, Women's Health, PR Week,* Forbes Health, *Delicious Living, Chicago Tribune, The Detroit News, Atlanta Journal-Constitution, SHAPE,* WCBS-TV, CNN iReport, *Daily Mail,* and *The Sunday Times.*

She also has written articles and op-ed pieces for numerous publications and websites, including www.HealYourLife.com, www.SheKnows.com, www.eDiets.com, and www.HuffingtonPost.com.

A lifelong learner, Connie trained with the Institute for Integrative Nutrition (IIN), iPEC Coaching (formerly the Institute for Professional Excellence in Coaching), and Northwestern University's masters in journalism program. She also studied with EFT Universe, the Brave Thinking

Institute, Tony Robbins, Marci Shimoff, Jack Canfield, Deepak Chopra, and Mel Robbins.

Connie loves to dance to music, take daily bicycle rides or long walks by the ocean, do Pilates, read or listen to audiobooks, play tennis or pickleball, study transformation, and pen provocative essays. She lives in San Diego, where she strives to be better and better every day in every way.

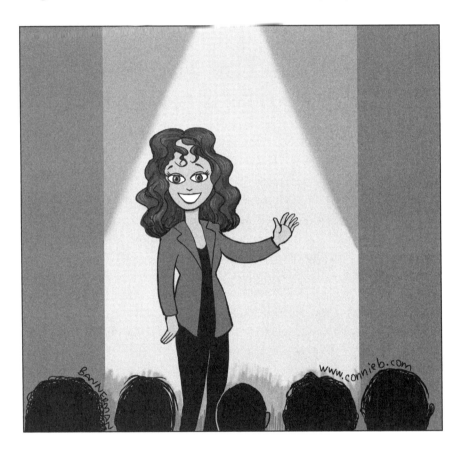

About the Recipe Developers
LIZETTE and GEOFF MARX

Lizette and Geoff Marx are professional holistic chefs, certified nutrition consultants, and culinary nutritionists. Lizette is a curriculum developer and instructor at Bauman College Holistic Nutrition and Culinary Arts in Berkeley, California, and a program coach at the Academy of Culinary Nutrition in Toronto, Ontario, Canada. The culinary couple teaches and promotes healthy, anti-inflammatory cooking methods, which are the best for your long-term health and vitality. All of their recipes embrace the healing qualities of SOUL (Seasonal, Organic, Unrefined, Local) food. www.marxculinary.com

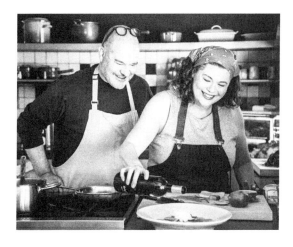

About the Cartoonist
ISABELLA BANNERMAN

Isabella Bannerman is the Monday artist for "Six Chix," a comic strip that is internationally syndicated by King Features. Isabella's award-winning cartoons and illustrations have appeared in many publications, including *The New York Times*, *Glamour*, and *Funny Times*. Isabella also has done animation work on MTV's "Doug," "Pee Wee's Playhouse," MTV spots, and other television shows and commercials. Her work has been recognized by the National Cartoonists Society, The Newswomen's Club of New York, and the Newseum. www.isabellabannerman.com

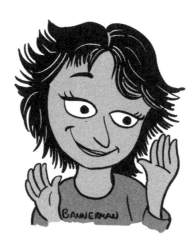

NOW WHAT?
Your Next Steps to
Bounce Back Boldly

Now that you finished this book, what do you do next? After all, additional challenges may come up. The good news is that you now have an array of fast, easy, convenient tactics to help you stretch, grow, and Bounce Back Boldly. In addition, I'm here to support you to make positive, lasting changes to your health, waistline, mindset, and life.

Here are additional ways I can continue to help you:

- **You can join my Bounce Back Boldly Bootcamp:** To go deeper into the material I share in this book, I invite you to join my companion bootcamp. When you participate in this program, you get my personal help to identify why you blew your diet, Crush Your Cravings, clear blocks to success, and tackle your cherished dreams and goals. Learn about my course by visiting www.BounceBackBootcamp.com.

- **Connect with me:** Let's stay in touch! I love hearing from readers. E-mail me links to interesting articles, interviews, ideas, books, or studies. Ask me questions to answer on my blog. Sign up for my weekly ezine.

www.connieb.com
www.bouncebackdiet.com

Let's Get Social!

www.facebook.com/conniebennettfans
www.instagram.com/conniebennettauthor
www.x.com/smarthabitsgirl
www.linkedin.com/in/conniebennett/

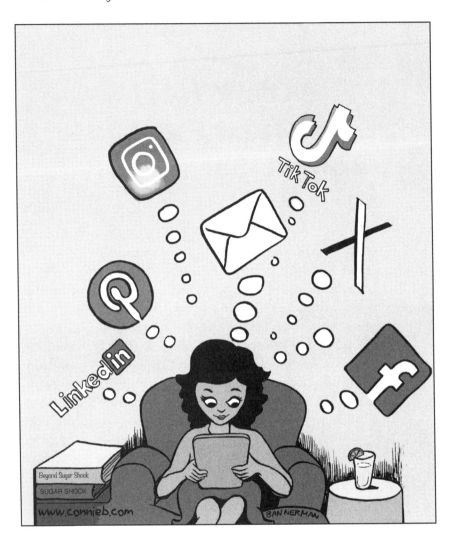

Please Share the Book Love!

If you liked this book, please tell your friends, loved ones, co-workers, fans,
and social media followers to buy one or more copies. Thank you so much in advance!
Gratefully, Connie